TEST TUBES
AND
DRAGON SCAL

This is a fascinating account of life in China i
1930's, as seen through the eyes of a young Amer
in the ancient Szechuan city of Chunking on th
China's richest, most powerful and romantic po
Chinese medicine and anxious to learn more abo
to supervise a Chinese hospital and is plunged i
exotic world both medieval and modern, where
coolies and rickshaws mix with the rising milita
soon overtake the country. As he learns more
Chinese remedies, Basil is drawn into the turbule
period, treating Generalissimo Chiang Kai-shek
conflict between the Communists and the Central
he goes on his medical rounds, treating patients
Chinese methods including *feng shui* with his o
fully into the life of the city, traveling the river by s
in markets, watching fortune tellers, entering
friendships and, through medicine, gaining intima
the heart of the Chinese character, and into the com
internal politics that would shortly erupt into war.
insightful comparisons between the health of Chine
people. Vivid prose brings the city and its
complimented by delightful line drawings.

TEST TUBES
AND
DRAGON SCALES

GEORGE C. BASIL

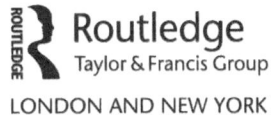

Routledge
Taylor & Francis Group

LONDON AND NEW YORK

First published in 2006 by
Kegan Paul International

This edition first published in 2010 by
Routledge
4 Park Square, Milton Park, Abingdon, Oxon OX14 4RN
605 Third Avenue, New York, NY 10017

*Routledge is an imprint of the Taylor & Francis Group,
an informa business*

British Library Cataloguing in Publication Data
A catalogue record for this book is available from the British Library

Publisher's Note
The publisher has gone to great lengths to ensure the quality of this reprint
but points out that some imperfections in the original copies may be
apparent. The publisher has made every effort to contact original copyright
holders and would welcome correspondence from those they have been
unable to trace.

ISBN 13: 978-0-7103-1209-9 (hbk)

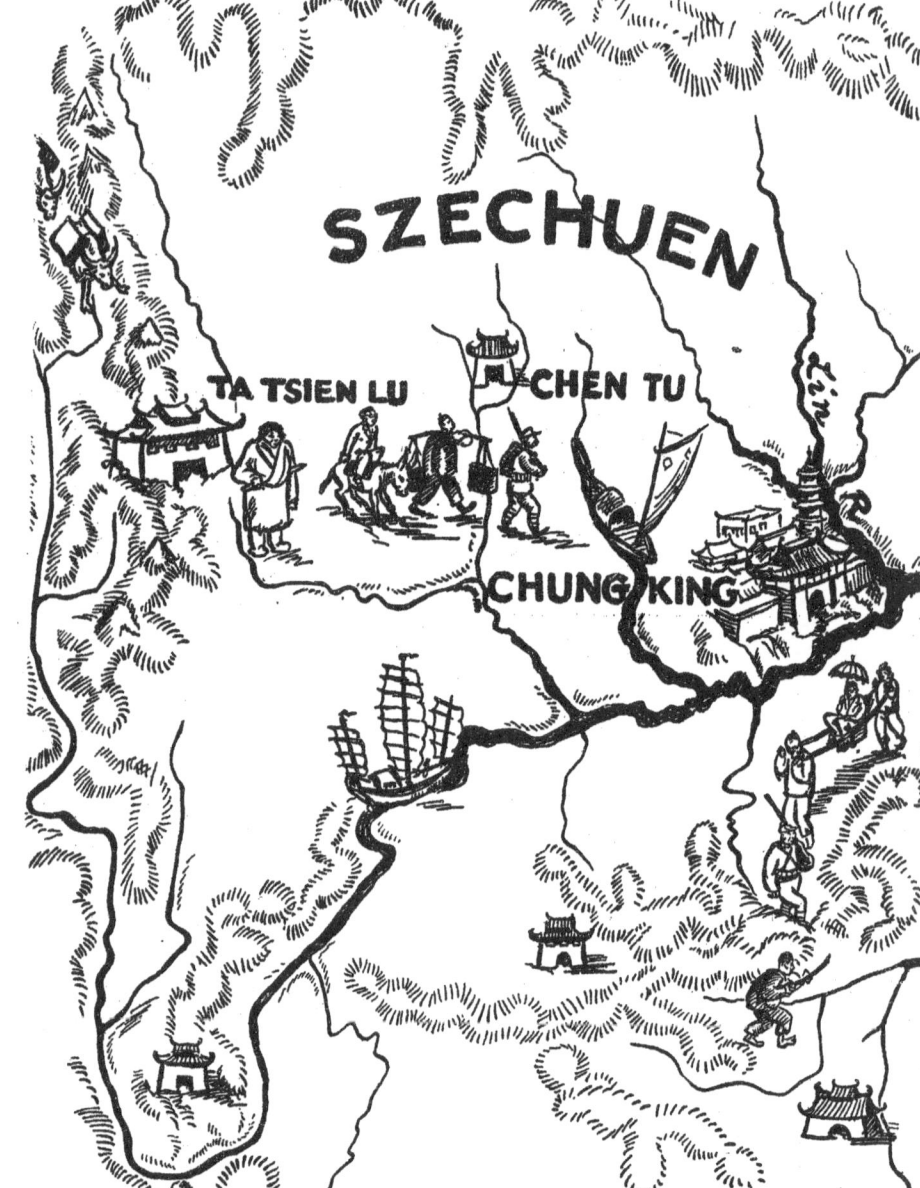

SZECHUEN

TA TSIEN LU   CHEN TU

CHUNG KING

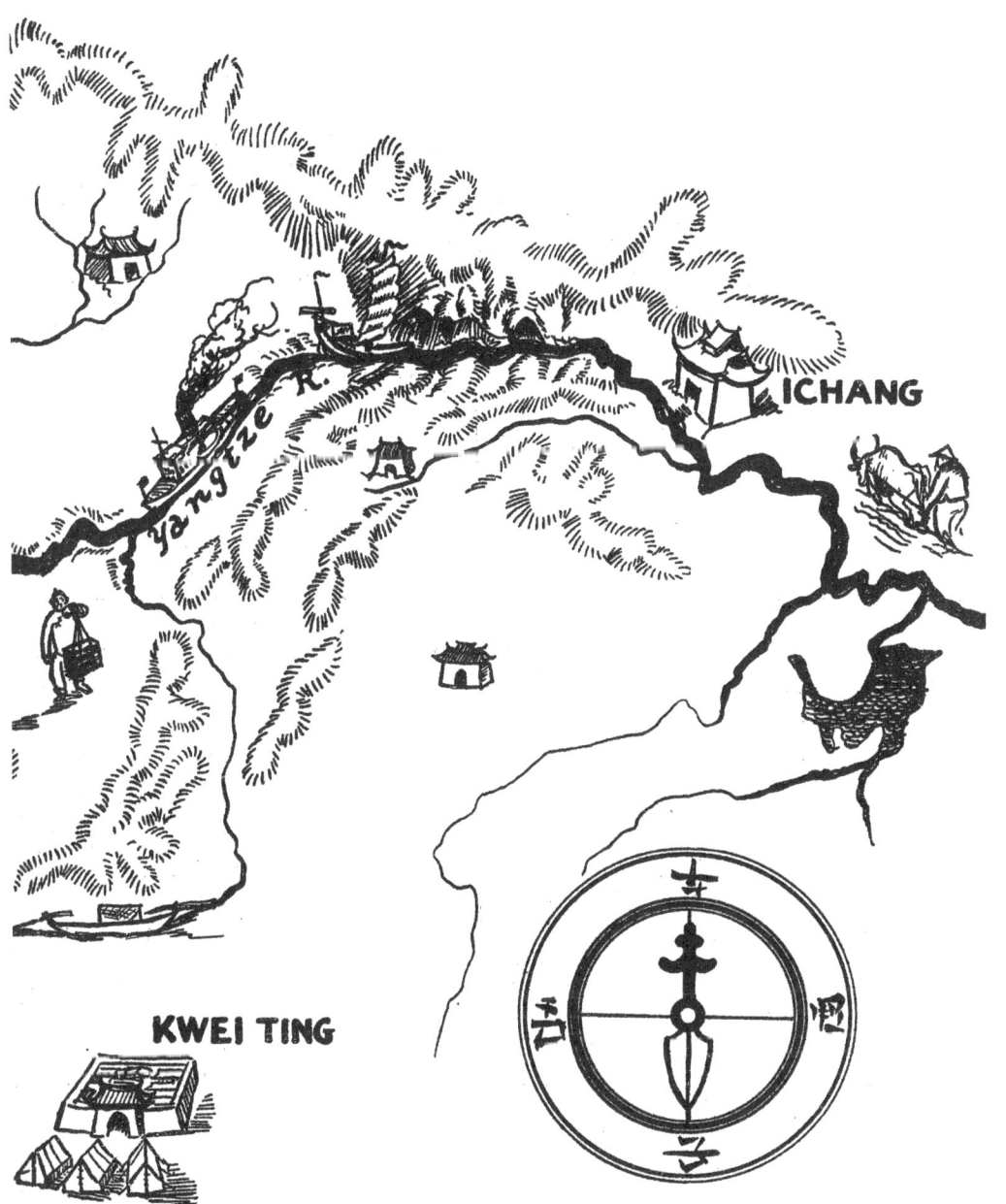

ICHANG

KWEI TING

To the memory of my mother,
MARGARET PURDY BASIL,
this book is humbly dedicated.

All names in this manuscript
are fictitious.

The Authors

FOREWORD

This book is the story of an American doctor's activities within the ancient walls of Chungking, a city deep in the unfathomable heart of the Orient.

Founded (according to historical tradition, in 2200 B.C.) on a rocky peninsula at the confluence of the Lin and Yangtze rivers, Chungking early became a rich prize, for possession of which men were to fight almost unceasingly throughout the centuries. During four thousand years of conflict, of annual floods, and of devastating fires, this prosperous port and financial center of Szechuen Province clung stubbornly to its ancient pattern of existence. It was not until the nineteen-thirties, when the Central Government decided on Chungking as national capital, that the city was forced to bridge the gap between its beginnings and the present day.

Through the ages, China's traditional capitals, Loyang, Peking, and Nanking have symbolized romance to the average citizen of the world. This latest one had neither beauty nor glamour to offer; instead it was ugly, filthy, and crowded beyond expression. The two rivers swirled muddily about its base, and clouds of mist during most of the year veiled its heights from the sun. The climate was so unpleasant as to defy description; and yet, in spite of all these handicaps, Chungking had always possessed a rare and mysterious ability to bind men to her.

Further proof of the city's spell is to be found in the pages of this personal history, as Doctor Basil related it to me. When for the last time his sedan-chair descended the flights of steps from the Tai Ping Gate to the Yangtze, Chungking looked much the same as it had for a thousand years or more. Today this picture has been transformed; but at the best, airports, broad highways, and public utilities accomplish only superficial changes. Somewhere beneath the concrete, the twisted cables, and the incongruous whirring of Occidental machinery pulsates the same disturbing personality that has made Chungking through the ages one of China's richest, most powerful, and most romantic ports.

With cities, as with men, individuality lies among the imponderables and, in this case, beyond the reach of Japan's ability to bomb or burn. Today, as fast as destruction occurs, men rebuild. Should the last tiled roof crumble to fragments and the last citizen flee, it seems unlikely that Chungking, with her feet set on rock and the roots of her vitality deep in men's memories, will share for long the fate of those other cities that are buried in history's pages.

March, 1940
Briar Cliff on Severn   ELIZABETH FOREMAN LEWIS
Arnold, Maryland

TABLE OF CONTENTS

Marginal illustrations
based on sketches
made in China by
RAYMOND CREEKMORE

CHAPTER I

The Man with a Plow

"Chungking was bombed again today." With somber regularity my morning paper reports these air attacks as I start the day's round of patients here in my Annapolis office. The city's utilities, I am told, rendered temporarily useless time after time have been promptly returned to public service. At the siren's first signal, "All clear!" the engineer corps remove debris and repair the gaping shell pits in the broad new motor roads. Few military or industrial objectives have been seriously damaged. Whether the short, stocky invaders playing their game of death so gaily in the sky are just poor marksmen or whether they find themselves unable to resist destroying schools, hospitals, and refugee camps, it is difficult to decide. However that may be, it is these benevolent institutions, residential districts, and the modern steel and plate-glass business section that lie in smoldering ruin; while the American Hospital, as yet miraculously unharmed, is filled to capacity with the shattered bodies, not of soldiers, but of helpless civilians.

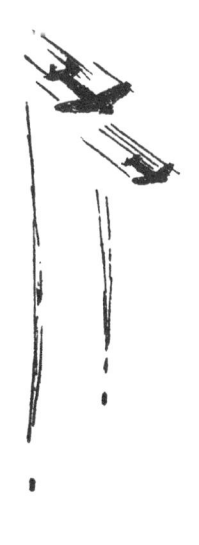

1

With mention of the hospital, this cumulative record of suffering and destruction becomes most real to me, for every part of that building is as familiar to my memory as is any of the medical equipment I have here at hand in Maryland. It is the references to motor roads, modern structures, and public utilities that bewilder me.

I am, it is true, seven years and ten thousand miles distant from Chungking, but when I left there in 1932, the city was almost the same as it had been for twenty centuries or more. Population remained numerically static around the half-million mark. Citizens were quite content to have their native place recognized as one of China's great ports; they considered it vastly superior to the provincial capital of Szechuen, which was Chengtu, three hundred miles away.

At that time the Chungkingese, arrogant and self-sufficient in their isolation, would have scoffed at the suggestion of ever becoming closely involved with the Chiang Kai-shek government, then centralized at Nanking. To their own province they paid only lip-service loyalty; to any authority outside its boundaries they were openly and vociferously antagonistic. That by 1939 their numbers might increase to a million and one half would have been a more acceptable idea, though even the most complacent among them could hardly have considered such enormous growth within the realm of probability.

Public utilities did not then exist, excepting a newly installed water system, which most inhabitants refused to patronize, much preferring the old methods of buckets filled from the Yangtze's muddy current and carried by man-power to their doors. Coolies delivering this commodity rubbed shoulders with others whose loads of sewage were headed for the fields.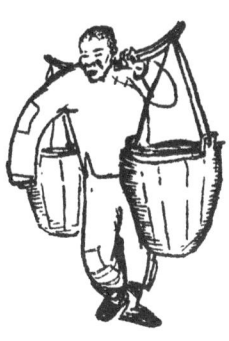

Most shops were of wood or plaster and open-fronted to the street, with only wooden grillwork to separate their counters from the passing throngs. People walked, or rode in sedan-chairs up and down the same narrow flights of stone steps as had their ancestors for several thousand years. To try to link modernity with the city that I knew, seems as fantastic as to attempt a description of life on Mars. And yet, in seven short years, this very miracle, I understand, has been achieved.

Difficult as it is to accept Chungking's physical changes, I find it even harder to think of the place as the present capital of all China and also as a gigantic clearing house for sixty million refugees. Uprooted from homes centuries old along the coast, the Yangtze Valley, and the North China plain, these men, women, and children, their families scattered and possessions gone, trek the endless miles toward Szechuen and the hinterland beyond that life may be started anew.

The Chinese have a proverb: "There is no grief so bitter as that for a dead heart," and these refugees on the march must know well the truth of that saying.

A Chinese clings forever to the bit of soil on which he and his ancestors were born, permitting himself to be torn from it only when Life and Death seem already to have done their worst. Through flood, drought, famine, plague, and civil strife, he remains in his accustomed location; if forced to flee, he knows no peace until return has been achieved. This racial devotion to place is difficult for the restless, roving-footed Westerner to understand, but it is the natural way of these Sons of Han.

Once during the Lantern Festival in Chungking I heard a prominent citizen say, "At home some of our customs for the Feast of Lanterns are very different from these."

Since the speaker's whole family was closely involved with provincial affairs, I asked in surprise, "B—— *Hsien-seng* (Sir), isn't Szechuen your home?"

"No—Shantung," the answer came in all seriousness. "My people moved here only four hundred twenty years ago."

In the only active military experience of my China residence, I was privileged to see this characteristic Chinese tenacity magnificently embodied in an old, blue-clad farmer driving his water buffalo before him at the plow. There could hardly have been a less auspicious occasion for noting spiritual values, nor was I in what might be called a receptive mood; yet the incident exerted an influence on my personal attitude

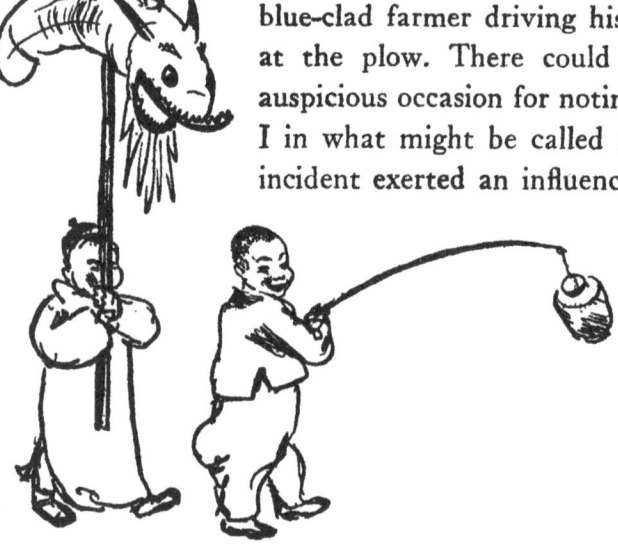

toward the Chinese that was out of all proportion to its size.

I was still comparatively new to the Chungking berth, with work, language study, and the countless adjustments to an alien world crowding my days, when an urgent business errand arose that necessitated a hurried trip to Shanghai. Due to the double expenditure of time and money, this journey of fifteen hundred miles by water was never undertaken lightly, and in my case disinclination was added to the other objections.

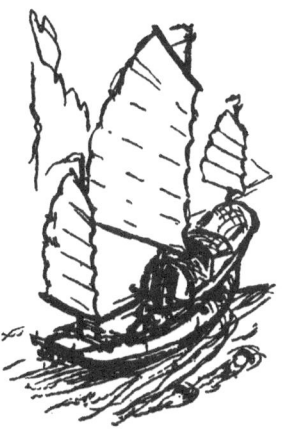

However, the trip through the Gorges went swiftly enough. We stayed on deck from dawn till dark, anxious to miss no single item of the constantly unrolling film of rapids, whirlpools, and towering cliffs. Frequently, small boats in a race with death dashed across the river before our bow, attempting to cut off any evil spirits that might be on their trail. Junks lay beached below all the great rapids, their water-logged cargoes spread on the shores to dry. When one calculated the enormous toll of life demanded by this river, it was not difficult at night, anchored in some small cove between walls of solid rock and listening to the water's unceasing hungry roar, to imagine the reality of these demons in which the Yangtze boatmen implicitly believed.

In Ichang we received our first setback. There, word awaited us that Communist troops were advancing

2

overland toward that port. Their course, it was reported, held pretty well to the north river bank, and it was likely that we should meet them the second or third day on the way to Hankow.

The Yankee skipper on our steamer, who had already had several unpleasant skirmishes with the Revolutionists, refused to risk his ship, and announced that he would return promptly to Chungking. Accustomed to occasional bandit assaults, most Upper River steamers had thin armor plate on the most vulnerable points. In warding off stray shots this was quite satisfactory; it was not meant, though, to withstand heavy fire.

When the captain learned shortly afterwards that a gunboat would be sailing around the hour of his own posted departure and would see the steamer through the dangerous district, he changed his mind again and decided to continue to Shanghai. "I just hope that those beggars take a few pot shots at us *this trip*," he told me with a calculating glint in his eye. "Last time they picked off one of my Chinese crew—he was a good fellow, had been with me for years—and I'd like nothing better than to see them swallow a dose of their own medicine."

He was not to be disappointed, for trouble occurred the second afternoon out of Ichang. In this narrow section of the Yangtze the ship following the channel was only about thirty yards from shore. The long, broad dike on the northern bank was decorated, oddly enough it seemed to me, with small red flags placed at regular intervals. My American background had taught me to look on red flags as workmen's warning signals, and I supposed in this case they had been placed on the dike for that specific purpose.

The officers, fortunately, recognized these small ensigns for what they were and ordered all passengers immediately to the armored enclosure. Simultaneously with this command, the dike, which a moment earlier had shown no signs of being occupied, now came alive with armed troops; and a rain of bullets began spattering the steamer.

All day the gunboat had been following us slowly, and the word that it was now coming into sight created a feeling of relief aboard the steamer. Ordinarily in the face of such fire our captain would have had only one recourse—full steam ahead. Instead, as the gunboat "hove to," he slowed down, moving as close to the South Shore as was possible in order that the other ship might slip between us and the Reds. The approach of the naval vessel presented a complication on which, I imagine, the Communists had not counted. A moment or so later the rumbling of three-inch shells accompanied the sharper explosions from machine guns and rifles.

Through a narrow window I watched this engagement. At the very beginning I had noticed in a field beyond the dike an elderly farmer plowing with a water buffalo. My first thought was that someone should force the old fellow to hunt a safer spot, but just how this message was to be conveyed I had no idea. Afterwards I realized how futile such an effort would have been. The exchange of fire was now incessant. Many of the small red flags were already down, together with a number of the human beings who had placed them there, and it seemed hardly likely that the plowman and his beast of burden could escape being hit.

When the first curtain of smoke and dust cleared, I saw with relief so deep it surprised me, that he was still standing beside his animal, motionless as if lost in wonder at the foolishness of man. Apparently he had no idea of seeking safety elsewhere; his job was to till this strip of ground, and by remaining, he declared to Heaven and Earth his intention not to be swerved from that purpose. Even before the next cloud screened him from me, he had begun again to drive rhythmically up and down the small field, turning furrows no different, I judged, from those made in an hour of peace.

Meanwhile men of his own race continued to fight with outsiders on a ship, for reasons that were obscure to him. The outcome of this strife probably concerned him little—these revolutionists were as foreign to his tradition as were the pink-skinned barbarians aboard the vessels. They were equally guilty of the folly of war, which, as the Sages had always taught, was the most wasteful of all pursuits. Even the babes under his roof knew that man's first duty was to labor and be strong; the second, to produce and rear his own kind to the honor of their ancestors. Nothing more was required. What did worry him at the moment was that the ground might suffer—to tear up fields that meant life to him and his neighbors—*ai*, that was an evil for which he had no words!

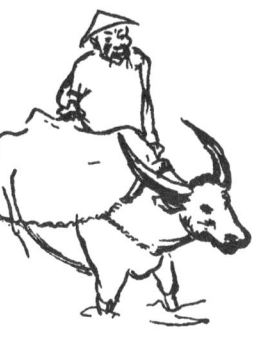

The shell fire was by this time proving too heavy for the troops on the dike; they now broke ranks and dashed wildly across the open fields, making themselves perfect targets had the gunboat been interested in anything more than teaching the offenders to respect unarmed passenger steamers. I was afraid that trampling feet might succeed where shot and shell had failed, but the plowman must have borne a charmed life, for he was still standing when I next saw him.

With the battle over, the steamer now churned slowly back into the channel, and passengers returned to decks. The dike, dotted with fallen flags and still, crumpled figures, was badly damaged and would need extensive repairs before late summer rains made the Yangtze a threat. Shell holes gaped in the once level fields, and a clump of bamboos, the only trees in sight, had been sheared of their tops. Farmer, buffalo, and plow, these alone remained unchanged.

Thinking the usual trite things about war's capacity for causing desolation, I glanced up to see the first mate beside me. "Looks as if a good many of those poor devils paid for their daring," I said.

"They got just exactly what they deserved," he told me flatly. "What beats me is how that old farmer managed to escape."

"That puzzled me too. You know he's been right there from start to finish."

He nodded. "They're a queer lot; nothing seems to feaze them." Tilting his cap, he scratched at the grizzled hairs that lay on his forehead. "Been on this Yangtze River twenty years; before that I had a Foochow run, and I don't know 'em a bit better than when I first came out. I often wonder what they get out of life."

"Perhaps if they told us we wouldn't understand what they were talking about," I suggested half to myself.

He paused in readjusting his cap to eye me shrewdly. "Maybe you hit the nail on the head there. Well," he concluded, moving off, "whatever it is, they certainly work for it."

Receding in the distance, the plowman, outlined against the sunset, seemed, I thought, a symbolic figure of his people's ability to rise above adverse circumstances. Steadily turning under the blood-stained clods, he offered to his small, war-torn world the hope of life to be renewed in springing green.

Today one of Japan's thinly stretched lines of occupation includes on my map that Central China field, and it seems quite likely that the old farmer, if still alive, has been forced to flee with the others from his stricken district. I find myself wondering if he too is on the way to Chungking, or if he has already arrived there and been sent on to farther fields of work especially prepared in advance to receive him and all other homeless refugees.

In 1931, when I was in Chungking, the Central Government at Nanking, fully aware that Japan meant to force eventual war on China, took the first steps toward winning Szechuen's loyalty to the Chiang Kai-shek regime. Strategically entrenched beyond the Yangtze Gorges, this "Province of Four Streams" possessed not only the farthest of the river ports, but was itself the gateway to several other sparsely settled provinces. In these districts rich and unlimited resources had hardly been touched through the centuries. In the event of conflict, if Japan blockaded the coast and captured important Eastern cities as her admittedly superior mechanized forces seemed certain to do, it was clear that China's government, as it retreated slowly westward, could settle down in this hinterland and hold out indefinitely against the invaders. To commit Szechuen, though, to anything but her own narrow interests was an almost superhuman task, and it was accomplished only after the Generalissimo in person, with a well-chosen entourage, paid the province a prolonged visit.

With Western loyalty "in the bag," official and cultural China began moving in that direction immediately after the Japanese-arranged incident at Marco Polo Bridge opened the war in July, 1937. Industrial machinery, university equipment, state records, art treasures, and libraries were now gradually transported from endangered locations to safer ones near Chungking. By November, 1938, when that city became the accredited capital, it was already functioning politically, industrially, and educationally as the center of National Government.

The most urgent problem facing China's leaders, aside from the promotion of war itself, was to open up the other western provinces to the ever-increasing hordes of refugees from the coast. As all roads had once led to Rome, so now all China roads led to Chungking, and modern highway construction became the most important of all goals. Limitless in man-power and flaming with patriotism, this united people has achieved miracles, and at this writing stands with its back to the Central Asian ranges, entrenched against the world.

Meanwhile the bombs continue to fall. In such destruction, I ask myself, how does the youth, Lu Dih-dih, handicapped by that stiff-swinging leg, find shelter in time? What of the chair-coolies on whose stout shoulders I learned to know Chungking—do they perhaps carry the wounded? What of the militarists and officials who once added exciting complications to my days? What of the friendly merchants and street vendors? All the men, women, and children that streamed through the hospital's doorways have become my fresh concern. For it is to these people that I owe my debt; together they helped me to discover for myself the wisdom and the mystery that have been Chungking's throughout the ages.

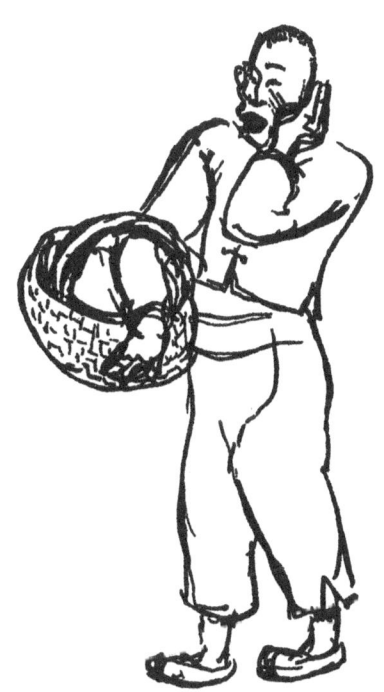

CHAPTER II

"Even the Gods Find It Difficult to Distinguish Between Pills, Powders, and Plasters" (Proverb)

How I personally happened to become connected with the Chungking scene is never to be explained with any degree of clarity. I can still hear my wife's first question about the appointment: "Why did you choose the Chungking Hospital rather than one in North or Central China?"

And my brief answer: "I want to work in the interior, not near the coast."

I knew little about the city save that it was fifteen hundred miles inland, was the one port to all West China, and that the hospital in question was reputedly large. For that matter, it was equally obscure why Maud and I should be in China at all, when we had fully expected to spend our lives in that mixture of Georgian architecture and historical tradition known to the United States Navy as "Crabtown," and to the rest of the world as Annapolis. The mere fact that three months earlier I had happened to find a travel pamphlet on a train seat seemed an absurd explanation. Yet that was all there was to offer. For the pages contained a

14

colored illustration of an American doctor disembarking from a small motorboat at an inland Chinese village, and as I studied it, the tides of envy surged within me.

That man, I told myself, was having a golden opportunity to see far-distant corners of the earth and at the same time to engage in almost single-handed combat with organisms that rarely if ever made their appearance in European or American test tubes. I left the booklet on the train, but the picture was printed on my mind. Later, as I stepped out into Baltimore's downtown traffic, I continued to remember a sluggish yellow stream, thatched huts, and cultivated terraces; naked babies, water buffaloes, and underslung hogs; and in their midst the incongruous foreign figure in white ducks and pith hat.

The thought of these led directly to local libraries, and what I found on the subject of Chinese medicine only whetted my interest. In China, I was informed, the profession was usually hereditary. Doctors felt no compulsion to share what they had learned with the rest of the world; instead, they jealously guarded their books of prescriptions until some close member of the family, preferably a son, was ready to start his career. With these the young medico set up shop; he needed nothing else, since neither certificate nor license was required for establishing a practice.

Chinese tradition was stoutly opposed to any disfigurement of the body after death; adding point to this attitude was the punitive custom of mutilating criminals following execution. Accordingly, the doctor was given no opportunity to study anatomy through dissection. Women patients never had physical examinations as we know them. The physician carried with him a doll-like feminine figure a few inches long. Sometimes these little figurines were beautifully made of ivory, though usually they were of cheaper material crudely carved. On the doll the patient pointed out just where her own pain occurred, and from that a diagnosis was made.

Chinese materia medica was highly interesting; it was as often startling. I learned from the Frenchman, Du Halde, in his book, *The Art of Medicine Among the Chinese*, written in 1735, that ginseng and tea were indispensable ingredients of almost every prescription; animals and herbs contributed most of the other essentials. Large white ants powdered with tea seeds and inhaled would clear up head noises. Ashes from burned elephant's flesh mixed with oil cured scalp sores. The ashes from the animal's breastbone acted as a tonic, and even more surprising, would help a man to swim. The ashes from a camel's chin whiskers cured internal hemorrhoids; the same beast's dried and powdered dung would stop nosebleed and kill vermin.

In most accounts there was a large section devoted to the subject of birth. Advice was so diverse as to recommend that a pregnant woman carry a dead sea horse in her garments to insure easy delivery, and that horse-radish be used for cauterizing the umbilical cord.

At first reading a good many of these statements seemed as nonsensical as were the charms and incantations used by their priests for the same purpose—healing the sick. As I read on, though, surprises came thick and fast. I learned that the Chinese theory about the heart's connection with circulation had antedated Harvey by a thousand years or two. For centuries they had been applying the brain of a mad dog to the wound the animal had inflicted—a long way on the road to the Pasteur treatment. On cancerous flesh they laid slices of putrid pork, hoping that the worms in the meat would devour those hidden in the wound. What was the result of this therapy, I do not know, but modern medicine uses something of the same idea in placing blowfly maggots on wounds that refuse to heal. They taught the rest of the world how to inoculate against smallpox long before vaccination was discovered and accepted; and if European medicine had not been so self-sufficient, China might have added ephedrin, liver, pig's stomach, and bufagin to the list of Western drugs ages before they became popular remedies.

It soon became clear that many of those early Chinese physicians had built soundly enough; but superstition, like a slimily scaled dragon straight from China's imagination, had been permitted to crawl over the entire structure and blot out the light. A foreign doctor might learn much from this ancient system, though in order to do so, he would first have to scrape strenuously at scales. At the moment, my enthusiasm failed to consider that simply putting into use the little I had learned about *modern* methods might be a full-time job. It remained for Chungking and the future to enlighten me on that score.

So, with no sounder motivation than a picture in a travel booklet and a few items about Oriental medicine, I turned my back on all previous plans to practice my profession at home; and on a midday in May, after almost two months of travel, my wife and I looked through a haze of heat and sulphurous smoke across the water to Chungking.

Built high on tier after tier of a rocky peninsula formed by the meeting of the Yangtze and the Kialing, or the "Great" and "Little" rivers, as they are called locally, the city presented, from the lowest strata of huts perched on bamboo stilts above the mud to the highest spot on its ancient gray stone wall, a dilapidated, down-at-the-heel appearance. The swift, muddy current between us and the shore was alive with dirty houseboats and sampans, whose unkempt, ragged crews, competing for the steamer's business patronage, worked feverishly—jostling, shouting, screeching like a mob of scarecrows abruptly come to infuriated life.

Constantly on this trip up the Yangtze we had heard Chungking described as a "dump" and "the end of

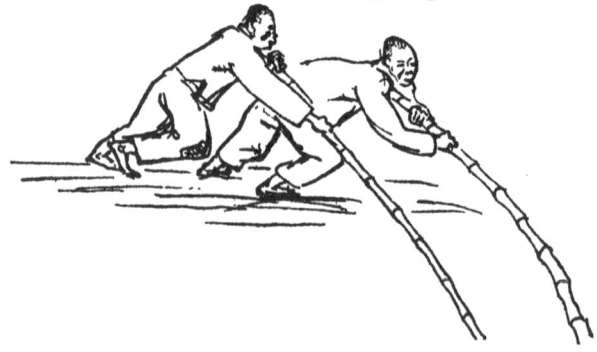

civilization." In spite of unfavorable epithets, I had
clung to my imaginative illusions concerning this far-
inland city. Now, faced by ugly reality, all my earlier
romantic notions about the port disappeared in the
smoky atmosphere. I had a sudden sharply distasteful
memory of a travel pamphlet. Why under heaven had
I let it help to persuade me to leave Maryland's
sunlit shores for the sake of working in this witch's
caldron of murk and filth?

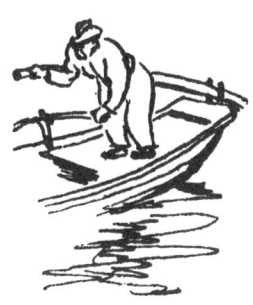

Next me at the rail a missionary who had boarded
the ship at Hankow, a thousand miles below, stood
making no effort to wipe away the tears that rolled
down her cheeks. Conscious of my attention, she
turned to explain brokenly, "The first sight of Chungking always does this to me."

I understood perfectly, until she added, "You get
so you wouldn't exchange it for any other place on
earth."

In response to a call, she now moved away, and I
stared after her with the same concentration ordinarily
given a specimen under the microscope. My gaze took
in again the noisy, stifling scene about me and that
builder's nightmare of mud, bamboo, and brick that
was apparently Chungking. "If ever a patient needed
to go under observation in a mental clinic," I told
myself solemnly, "that poor woman is one."

Maud had been exchanging gay farewells with the
officers and passengers; when in a moment of respite

she turned to me, her smile wavered. "The place looks pretty awful from here, doesn't it?" she whispered.

A hospital representative came aboard to welcome us and, appointing a servant to look after our baggage, he led the way to a waiting sampan in which we ferried to shore. There, coolies rushed to meet us with sedan-chairs, the indescribably filthy, closed variety to be hired on the streets.

"Would you rather walk or ride?" was the next question.

"Walk!" I answered, after one glance at the means of transportation.

In a midday temperature of 100° and a humidity striving to pass that mark, we started our climb up the hundreds of steps that led from the water-front to Chungking's city gate. It was a relief to pass at last from the glare into the shadows of the gateway. There we were accosted by guards and immediately surrounded by a curious group of hangers-on. Most of these we learned were soldiers disbanded weeks earlier by a local warlord. They had accommodated themselves to the heat by discarding most of their tattered uniforms and were now garbed only in trousers rolled to the thigh, straw sandals, and military caps with red bands.

While our companion discussed credentials with the city's protectors, I had time to glance about me, and the first sight was far from reassuring. In the public

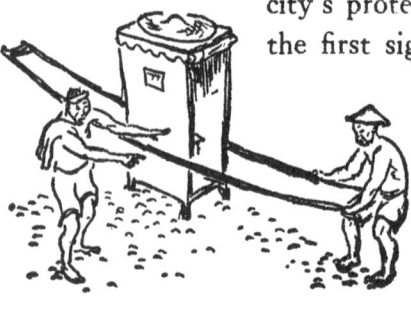

thoroughfare ahead, a passageway where a man could stand in the middle and touch either side with outstretched fingers, extended rows of gray stone steps. Here, I was to discover shortly, was a metropolis, which, limited in level expansion and crowded by an always increasing population, had chosen to go skyward endlessly on streets of stairs. Dirt-covered by centuries and time-worn by millions of human footprints, the depressions on some of these treads were deep enough to cradle a child's body.

Up and down, Chungking's life flowed in unceasing streams. Within these narrow lanes of progress the city steamed, and we climbed slowly, rubbing shoulders with the masses—rich and poor, old and young—most of them carrying on their faces or bodies the evidences of malnutrition, deformity, or disease. Slop carriers, their heavy buckets dripping malodorously on the slimy steps, crowded us to the wall; mangy, sore-infested dogs hampered our steps. In an occasional doorway a black, fly-blown sow nursed her thin litter, and everywhere bedraggled chickens blinked drowsily in their basket coops.

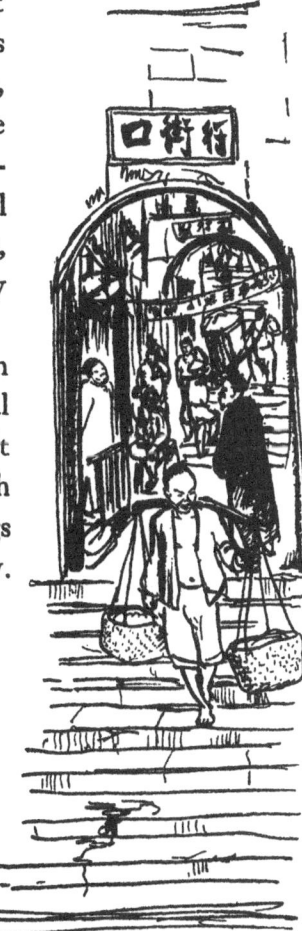

Tuberculosis, smallpox, trachoma, leprosy, skin infections, a host of other communicable diseases, all had left imprints on these human beings about us. It was exciting to imagine the possibilities in research that a bit of ooze from these steps or a few scrapings from a wall might offer a modern medical laboratory.

3

A hundred conversations beat on the ear at once, and, attempting without success to find a single familiar sound, I sensed for the first time the difficulties a veterinarian has with his patients. Would I ever learn any of this language? If not, I told myself dubiously, my work would be defeated at the start.

At an intersection a mob blocked our way. Curious, I peered over shoulders and noticed an angry guard standing above the battered body of a man. "What's happened?" I asked our guide.

"Probably beaten to death for stealing."

Fortunately my wife, still at the outer edge of the crowd, had seen and heard none of this. She was already beginning to look white from heat and fatigue, and I was relieved when our destination was finally reached.

We were, however, not permitted to stop there for long. A small reception planned for us out in the country necessitated another long, hot walk. When we finally got to bed that night, it was to toss restlessly for hours. Maud's first impressions of our new home had left her low in spirit, and my own mind held a good many questions.

Before leaving the States, I had been warned that in the Orient's unlimited field of opportunity two dangers lay in wait for the physician. The first was to labor far beyond his strength; the second, to lower standards of professional efficiency until usefulness was at a discount. Even if the language and all other difficulties should adjust themselves, was it still likely that one of these other pitfalls might prove my undoing? China's history testified to her uncanny ability in assimilating outsiders and their innovations. Who could say that after this ancient land had worked its will on me for several years, my own test tubes might not be encrusted with dragon scales?

Next morning we awoke to find ourselves victims of enteritis—our formal introduction to Chungking.

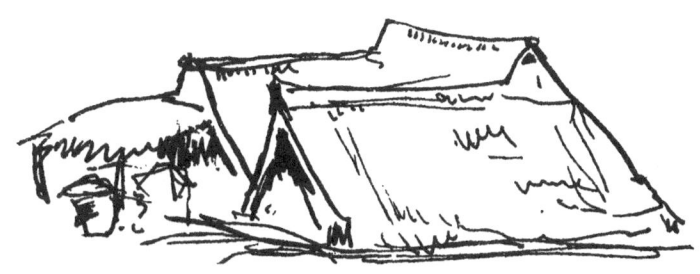

CHAPTER III

"To Become a Famous Doctor, a Man Needs to Know Little" *(Proverb)*

My first sight of the institution to which I had been appointed superintendent was one to be remembered. As we entered the stone gatehouse, several scrawny chickens and a pig hurried from our path. Never in my life had I seen anything like this coming from a hospital. A short stone walk led to the main building, where I found the same offensive odors as in the entrance, although the livestock was missing. Corridor walls were stained and spotted; and visitors, who seemed to be coming and going without supervision, spat on the floor at will.

"The place doesn't always smell like this, does it?" I asked, as my nostrils, searching for the familiar scent of anesthetics and antiseptics, were assaulted by a dozen others of decidedly questionable origin.

"If you stay in China awhile, you'll get used to that," my companion answered wryly.

"Not with my nose, I won't!"

"To attract these people as patients, they must first be made to feel at home, and that means compromising."

24

Silently I conceded the possible necessity of making some compromises in this alien environment, but with that overconfidence typical of the younger members of any profession, I determined that my compromises should not interfere with the fundamental principles of sanitation.

On our tenth day in Chungking we settled down to language study, and a week or two later crossed the Yangtze in the annual foreign exodus to the Hills for the period of Great Heat. These low-lying ranges south of the river had been hidden by murky atmosphere the day of our arrival on the *Wan Lu* and now afforded us a pleasant scenic surprise. A succession of graduated terraces used for the cultivation of peanuts, beans, and sweet potatoes climbed the slopes, their pattern repeatedly broken by small green lakes of rice plants. In the wilder, more inaccessible areas, rare flowers and shrubs colored the year from season to season.

Viewed from here, beyond water gleaming in the sunlight, even Chungking acquired a semblance of beauty. On clear days one could gaze over the southwestern ranges toward Kweichou and Yunnan provinces, then, giving rein to the imagination, cross the borders of Indo-China and Burma. That those same distant provinces, shrouded by centuries in mystery, would within a few years become the "Promised Land" for pioneering young China was something beyond the most active fancy.

Several times a week I commuted to the hospital in my first local purchase, one of the comfortable wicker sedan-chairs used by foreigners. Swinging along in the freshness of morning, with the chair-bearers chanting as their bare feet slapped the narrow paths between fields, I began to be infected by the Szechuen scene. After being ferried over the river's swift current, travelers faced the challenge of Chungking's endless stairs. The sedan, its cross poles resting on the coolies' shoulders, was now suspended at sharp angles in mid-air to meet the constant demands of ascending and descending slopes of progress. As I became used to this riding "on the bias," I found ample opportunity to study the crowds that pressed about me. Under the physical impact of this ancient civilization my interest quickened. Gradually I grew aware that while the Chungkingese might still seem much like guinea pigs for medical experimentation, they were fast becoming individual guinea pigs, each with characteristics and qualities all his own.

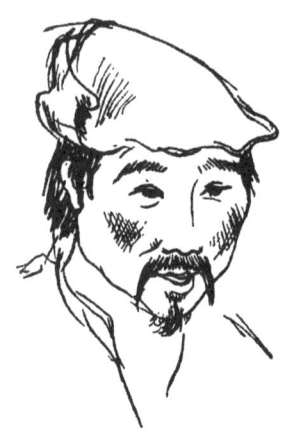

Faces that on the day of arrival held for my eye only ignorance and depravity now presented expressions of patience, courage, or cheerfulness, and sometimes all three. Honesty forced the admission that while I, as yet, had no real liking for these people, no longer were they to be dismissed in the blanket wave of repulsion I had first experienced. Here behind an exterior unfamiliar to me, man struggled stubbornly for continued existence under almost incredible hand-icaps.

One question I was to ask myself repeatedly was how these Chungkingese, confronted always by pestilence and poverty, managed to survive in such numbers. The correct answer probably lies hidden in the centuries of hardships their race has been called upon to endure. These, it may well be, have developed a resistance in the individual sufficient to discourage even the stoutest-hearted organisms bent on his destruction. The Chinese custom of consuming steaming hot food does much, of course, to counteract infections, though this protective insurance, I venture the theory, carries its own danger. In eating, the rice bowl is held close to the lips and with the chopsticks lumps of food are thrown swiftly to the back of the mouth. As time passed, I found myself treating a disproportionate number of people for malignant throat conditions, and these, I came to believe, were caused by the constant assault of hot objects on the soft palate.

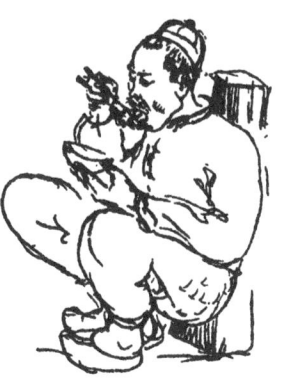

Slowly I was learning the ropes at the hospital and, incidentally, noticing peculiarities of custom and manner common to Chinese life and to the local practice of medicine in particular. Today, memory of the swiftness with which I adopted some of their ways makes me gasp. Only the sublime confidence of young manhood could have led me to "rush in where angels fear to tread."

I had been given to understand that "face"—prestige, reputation, or whatever you choose to call it —was the most important of all possessions among the Chinese. Ability and learning evoked their greatest respect and after these, physical age, for years were supposed to add knowledge through experience. As a newcomer, and much younger than any other medical worker in Chungking, I was faced from the start by the problem of overcoming these handicaps and of building a reputation out of something besides proven ability, which for purposes of immediate usefulness worked too slowly.

As it was, the Chinese themselves provided me with advertising weapons. According to *kwei-jui* (custom), one of the most powerful words in their language, courtesy demanded that one always discredit himself, his character and ability, his family and home, and at the same time praise the other fellow to the skies. In speech, the greatest men underestimated themselves the most, and I began to copy their ways by working overtime the accepted phrase, *puh gǎng däng* (most unworthy) in response to compliments paid to me.

When after a successful abdominal operation, the patient's friends insisted that I must know a great deal about the *tu tz* (stomach, or more inclusively in Chinese, the entire abdomen), I would reply, "Most unworthy! I know nothing at all about the *tu tz.*"

This method worked like too much yeast in buckwheat dough, for the more I discredited my efforts in speech the more the Chungkingese overrated my ability. I was soon in the impossible position of being considered an *all-round general specialist*. At first this absurdly devised reputation seemed harmless enough, and the strangeness of our new life with its increasing activities forbade my pondering too thoughtfully on the possibilities of repercussions. Only after a return to America had given me perspective on the Chungking scene, did I realize the part such nonsense had played in the creation of numerous difficult situations.

The first of these came early in my career. One midsummer afternoon just after I had finished a tonsillectomy and was scrubbing up to return to the Hills, Doctor Tu, the Chinese resident, sought me out to announce in his careful English, "*Beh Ih-seng* (Basil Doctor), General Chang is in the office and wishes to see you."

"Me?" I asked incredulously. "I thought all the officials patronized the other institution."

Doctor Tu smiled mischievously. "On the street at present one hears much talk about our own hospital. An official's ears are large; perhaps the General, too, has heard these rumors."

My collar felt uncomfortably tight as I went on scrubbing. "All right, I'll be out there in a few minutes," I promised briefly.

When my first flush of embarrassment had subsided, I began to feel that this caller might represent opportunity knocking at the door. For a long time the hospital had been catering almost entirely to the lower classes, and it was my opinion that a sprinkling of wealthy and important patients might prevent the budget's becoming the cause for headaches it now seemed to be.

To make a good impression was highly important. Since setting foot in Shanghai, I had been told again and again that a youthful appearance was a serious handicap in this land. To avoid this I had already grown a mustache. Now stepping into the small optical storeroom, I substituted a pair of large, horn-rimmed spectacles with unground lenses for my own less conspicuous ones. Chinese scholars invariably wore these to create an air of learning and dignity. Thus fortified, I assumed what I considered the blasé professional manner that might come from long experience in handling officials, then walked firmly down the corridor to the office.

It was slightly disconcerting to find the patient also using one of my chosen properties to enhance his own appearance, for the frames on *his* nose did not even contain lenses. He was about five feet, seven inches in height, with stocky body and smooth, well-shaped face. His hair was cropped short in typical Chinese fashion, and his garments, rich in material and simple in cut, were of native style in contrast to the foreign suits affected by many of the younger officials.

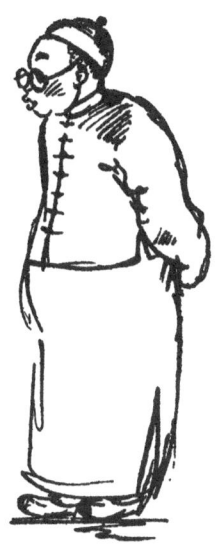

After an exchange of elaborate courtesies, with Doctor Tu acting as interpreter (since I had only a few Chinese phrases and the patient no English at all), it became clear that the visitor needed medical attention but wished no examination at the moment. The interview ended with a request that I call the following Friday morning at the General's residence in the Hills and there, when professional matters should be concluded, be his guest at a feast.

At eight o'clock Friday an ornate chair with bearers in official livery appeared before our bungalow, and I set off confidently on my first introduction to the Chinese official world. On arrival I was ushered into a large reception hall, where my patient provided an interpreter, then introduced me to a group of friends. In the center of the hall stood tables for the feast, laid with rare porcelain bowls and silver chopsticks and elaborately decorated with flowers. One chair was almost covered with floral designs, and recognizing this as the seat of honor and the doctor as the special guest on this occasion, I could see myself soon occupying that surprisingly elevated position.

"If General Chang is ready, I shall now examine him," I suggested to the interpreter, then waited for the crowd to grant us privacy before I began asking questions. No one moved.

"Please invite these others to leave!" I whispered to the go-between.

He glanced up in surprise. "They are the General's friends and he wishes them to remain."

This was a new wrinkle in medical practice, but, smothering further objections, I turned to the patient. Symptoms pointed superficially to nephritis (Bright's Disease) and with no laboratory test as guide, I decided to look at the eye-grounds for further proof. Slowly and carefully I began to explain that I must put drops in his eyes to dilate them; that these would blur vision, and for a number of hours he would not see clearly. "You understand what I am going to do?" I questioned.

"Yes, yes, Honorable Doctor!" came the reassuring response.

I still had my doubts. "You understand," I repeated, "that when you look at your fingers, you will not see them clearly? You may even see two where one was."

"Yes, yes!"

It seemed uncomfortably possible that the interpreter had not made the matter entirely clear, but I dropped a little homatrophine in each eye and waited for its effect in relaxing the iris. Suddenly my patient swallowed, looked startled, and spat on the floor. The drug was apparently working down to his palate. Almost immediately he began to realize that vision was blurring, then remembering the statement about fingers, he stared at a hand and discovered the worst. Fright

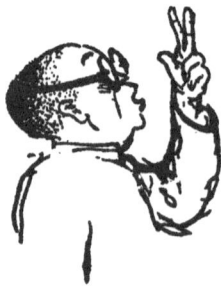

spread over his face, and by way of consolation I suggested, "Don't be alarmed! Your eyesight must become even more blurred before I can see what is wrong."

The effect of this speech was exactly contrary to hope. At once the General demanded, "Give me back my sight!" Next as the drug continued to act, he shouted, "I am poisoned! I can taste it on my tongue. This foreigner has killed me!" Rising to his feet, he called for his favorite wife, then crossed the room to kneel before a Buddhist altar in one corner. The wife appeared immediately (only an emergency could have justified this impropriety in a Chinese room where men were gathered for a serious purpose), and added feminine wails to the general bedlam.

"For heaven's sake tell them he's all right!" I appealed to the interpreter, after listening to his explanation of this astonishing activity. "Nothing's going to happen."

His statements fell on ears already deafened by angry, excited discussion, and the General's guests pressed so closely about us that their sibilant speech spattered me with saliva.

"Return General Chang's sight!" they demanded harshly.

"I can't yet."

"You took it away!"

"Yes."

"Then why can't you give it back?"

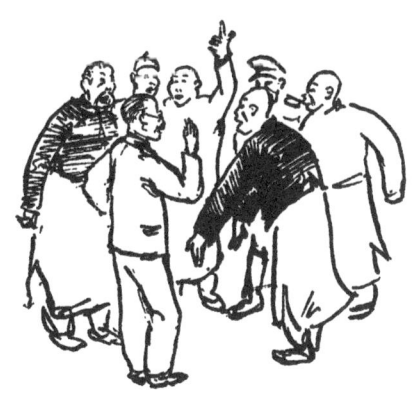

"A little patience! His eyes will be all right to-morrow."

"Tomorrow will not do! Heal the General's eyes at once, or we shall know it is true that you came here to blind and poison him."

"I am here for one reason only—to help a patient. Moreover, I came only at his personal invitation, and if it's just the same to you, I'll be going."

"Of a certainty, no!"

"Why not?"

"You may not leave until his sight is restored."

"I told you that may take a day, and I have important duties at the hospital."

"No one in all Chungking is more important than General Chang. You will remain here!"

Servants entered now and cleared the tables. A moment later I was led to another room and left there alone to cool my heels. When the interpreter finally joined me, I asked him, "Why did they put me in here?"

He coughed hesitatingly—no Chinese finds it easy to be rude. "When a man is sick, he prefers the companionship of old friends, *Beh Ih-seng.*"

I shrugged my shoulders impatiently. "Except for blurred vision, he hasn't any more wrong with him than before I came."

"Truly, Honorable Doctor, but in China we think it very bad fortune to be blind."

"But he's not blind! He merely cannot see clearly!"
The interpreter politely pondered these contradictions.
In this case explanations were futile; I muttered under
my breath.

"Excuse me! What did *Beh Ih-seng* say?"

The question was ignored. "Will you please tell
them again that there is nothing the matter with
General Chang? I can help him take a nap, if he would
like to rest a little; afterwards we can finish the examination." Sleep might quiet the patient's nerves and
make him more amenable to treatment, I decided.

This message was delivered promptly and the interpreter returned, accompanied by a spokesman for the
enemy. "By what method will you cause the General
to sleep?" was the next question.

I produced my hypodermic needle. Chinese medical
practice is so familiar with acupuncture that this small
instrument met with less objection than it might have
even at home; but on the point of acceptance, the other
paused.

"Suppose the drug in this is harmful?"

"If you wish," I interrupted, "I'll first use the
needle on myself."

The spokesman studied me gravely, then went out
to go into a huddle with his companions. A little later
the interpreter and I were invited to rejoin the crowd.

"Give yourself this medicine and let us see what
happens!" commanded the patient, who, completely

surprised at still being alive, was once more in command of the situation.

I put fifteen minims of sterile water in my arm, then walked around whistling a tune to indicate a physical well-being and a nonchalance I did not feel.

After watching me closely for a few minutes, the General agreed to take his own shot. I gave him one-half grain of morphine and almost before I could say, "Jack Robinson!" the head of Chungking was snoring on an ornate bench that graced the hall.

The patient must already have been exhausted from emotion, for it was surprising indeed to have the drug take effect so promptly on one who undoubtedly smoked some opium. This was my cue to show signs of drowsiness from my own hypodermic. I yawned broadly, then sitting down, leaned back with eyes closed and wondered unhappily how and when I was going to get out of this mess.

After what seemed an interminable period of inactivity, I decided that my simulated nap had served its purpose, came awake, and went over to the patient. He was breathing evenly as a baby. "You know that a poisoned man does not sleep so peacefully as that," I defended, in response to the questioning glances my action had aroused. Several indicated the wisdom of this point of view, and the atmosphere became slightly less frigid. "Now I must be going," I urged, "and tomorrow I'll return."

"No, the respected physician must wait until General Chang awakes." Courtesy dictated an addition which did not fool me for a minute, "The General will wish to thank *Beh Ih-seng*, himself."

Heavens, I asked myself with inward desperation, how long is that bird going to sleep? It was now noon-day and having had only a light breakfast to fortify me for this experience, I asked for a bowl of tea. This, in itself, was the most conclusive evidence of my present ostracism, for Chinese hospitality presses refreshments on a visitor at all hours. After the tea and another smoke I decided to risk waking the patient. As I had foreseen, his vision was temporarily clearer from sleep, and his spirits rose accordingly. He glanced about, murmured orders, and servants appeared to reset the tables. By the time this task was completed, the daylight to which his eyes had been exposed had done its unfavorable work, and sight blurred again. My host immediately barked out another command, and everything went off the tables once more, leaving me to occupy another Arctic island.

This was no longer even funny. Seething inside, I said in the calmest manner possible at the moment, "Permit me to go to the hospital, and I'll return with a drug to restore sight."

"No, Honorable Doctor, you must not spend so much energy. We will send a messenger in your place."

4

Grimly I wrote an order for some eserin and another note to Doctor Strobel, a medical free lance in Chungking and the one foreign physician who, I felt, might be of assistance in my predicament. His response was to arrive before the messenger with the drug. The official entourage welcomed him cordially, and after the usual ceremonial palaver, he made his way to my side and in a few sentences learned what had happened.

"We're going to have the devil of a time convincing these people of your helpful intentions," Strobel admitted gravely. "Every official in this country lives in constant fear of being poisoned by enemies. You're a foreign newcomer and here, after a few minutes in your hands, the most important man in the city at present suffers impaired eyesight." He paused, as I interrupted to say that I had done nothing uncommon to modern medical procedure, as he well knew.

"Yes, yes, I know," he acknowledged sympathetically, "but the Chinese don't—and you are lucky, indeed, not to have been treated more roughly than this."

When the messenger arrived with the drug, Doctor Strobel carefully explained to all concerned what I had been trying to do, and he assured them that I could improve the General's sight by putting a few drops of this new medicine in his eyes.

"No!" came the emphatic reply, and the suspicion previously limited to me now included Strobel as accomplice.

"I'll put some in my own eyes first," I offered.

After due consideration this concession was accepted, but before I could move, two of the City Fathers invited Strobel into another room for tea, insisting politely that he must not be troubled by these details.

"I'd insist on staying beside you if it would help," Strobel whispered. "If you need me, call out!"

"I'll be all right," I told him, not at all sure that I would, then I dropped some of the medicine in my eyes. Nothing happened, of course, so the patient submitted and in a few moments found his sight improved.

"Now," he asked in better humor, "please continue the examination."

"Your Excellency is tired. Permit me to return to the hospital at present and finish this tomorrow."

"Very well, but first we must eat a little."

Once more tables were set, and at five o'clock we sat down to the first real food that I had seen since breakfast. Doctor Strobel, reassured as to outcome, pleaded an ill patient as excuse for leaving before the feast. Although glad to eat, I was nevertheless uneasy, knowing that the eserin's effect would be limited in time. When the General began glancing again at his hands, the moment for another application seemed to have arrived.

"It's time to give you more drops!"

"Put them in your own eyes first!"

I complied, then treated his. The feast seemed to go on endlessly; much as I liked Chinese food, I could never recall afterwards what was served on that occasion. Since I couldn't keep putting eserin in his eyes forever, I acknowledged deep gratitude for this generous hospitality and again attempted farewells. The patient offered numerous objections.

"Your Excellency feels well now, is it not so?" I asked.

"True, but I wish the Honorable Healer to remain and talk a little."

I managed to convey the idea that nothing could possibly give me more pleasure, but having already overstayed my time, it would be more convenient to take advantage of this privilege some other day. "To be certain that you sleep well, permit me to help you again with a hypodermic."

"Give yourself one first!" the patient ordered with an amiable smile.

After repeating the earlier procedure, I was at last permitted to bow myself from the official presence. As the chair-bearers swung me across the Hills, the cool night air seemed more refreshing than any I had ever breathed. I directed the coolies straight to our bungalow and there I returned to spend a night in which sleep was broken by the recurring picture of my head on a bamboo spike outside the Chungking wall.

CHAPTER IV

The Barbarian Is Confronted by a Chinese Wall

Arriving early next morning at the hospital, I was told that a delegation from General Chang had been waiting there for an hour or two. The patient had awakened about four, as did most Chinese, and had sent at once for me to return and complete the examination.

"Have his eyes cleared yet?" I asked Doctor Tu.

"Still blurred, *Beh Ih-seng.*"

"Tell them I am extremely busy this morning and cannot spare time for a return to the Hills." Tu's surprised expression made me add a hasty account of the previous day's ordeal.

"He is a very important man—perhaps it might be wiser to grant his wish," ventured my Chinese assistant.

"Look, Tu, to quote your own proverb, 'Does the sensible goat willingly stick his head in the tiger's den'?"

Chinese humor came to the rescue. "Not if the animal wishes to live!"

"Well, that's the answer. I'll not call on that patient again, unless they haul me there in chains."

"He could do that, *Beh Ih-seng* understands?"

"Mnh!" I grunted. The General's power was not to be doubted. He had risen to his present position only through first being a ruthless warlord, and to have an unimportant foreigner meet with a fatal accident would not raise the international dither it might have even ten years earlier. To place myself in his hands again or to offend by refusal, seemed equally risky to me. Of the two I chose the second. "I'm not going, Tu. You may as well tell them now, so we can get on with our job."

But the delegation was not to be dismissed so easily. When Doctor Tu had explained most carefully that at present I must attend to very sick patients in the hospital, their spokesman demanded, "Which day then will *Beh Ih-seng* call?"

"Never!" I buzzed in Tu's ear.

"*Beh Ih-seng* feels that we can give better treatment if the General comes to the hospital."

"I don't want him here either," I protested sotto voce, but Tu, engaged in smoothing down the visitors, was paying no attention.

After some discussion, the callers bowed ceremoniously and departed. Curious, I asked, "How did you finally persuade them to go?"

"I told them, *Beh Ih-seng*, that you humbly appreciate the honor of serving so important a man. However, you have suffered from stomach trouble since arrival in Chungking and you must save strength by making the trip between the hospital and your home in the Hills only once a day. Therefore, if General Chang could come here, it would be better for both him and the doctor."

"Why didn't you suggest that they invite one of the more experienced Chungking physicians to look after him?"

"*Beh Ih-seng* expected me to offer such advice? *Ai-ya!*" Tu's eyes, under raised brows, now lighted with mischief, as he added, "True it is, no one of them would have dilated the eyes of a general with an army to command!"

Having no satisfactory retort to this, I remained silent. He next informed me that a generous sum had been left in the hospital office to pay for the previous day's visit.

Within a week or so, I received a number of elaborate gifts from the General. "What about these?" I demanded of Tu. "He has already paid more than the regular fee."

"A personal appreciation of your services!"

"So far I've been unable to do anything for that patient, and I refuse to be under obligation. Send them back!"

"To return them would be an insult."

"I won't keep them," I insisted stubbornly, "and that's final."

My Chinese assistant shrugged his shoulders over this delicate situation, but the gifts disappeared. Later I discovered they had been returned with a flowery note to the effect that the General had given the hospital far more than the usual charge, and it was beyond the bounds of generosity for him to send personal gifts as well. Were *Beh Ih-seng* to accept such magnificent and valuable articles, he would feel like a veritable earthworm, or its close relative, at least.

Several mornings afterward I was astonished by the appearance of General Chang and an interpreter at our Hills bungalow. Except for chair-bearers, these two were alone. Wondering what was afoot now, I assumed an air of courteous friendliness that matched the visitors' own and invited them into my study.

After a brief exchange of amenities, General Chang began to explain that his gifts to me had been an apology for acting so ungraciously that day in his home. "It is very hard for men who know only Chinese ways to understand foreign customs," he continued, then added, "I have heard that *Beh Ih-seng* thinks he was held prisoner—he was detained only to help my miserable self, had I needed assistance in recovering from the drug."

I could do nothing less than rise to the occasion, admitting that I was a witless newcomer and had completely misunderstood his intentions. Shortly afterwards, letting eye-grounds severely alone, I completed the examination so inauspiciously begun, and we parted most amicably.

"Permit me to call on you again, *Beh Ih-seng*," he said, stepping into his ornate chair.

"I shall be most unworthy of such honor! Any time I can serve Your Excellency, do not hesitate to let me know."

He turned again. "All the members of my council shall be examined!"

"This is too great a favor! Do you think twenty-five dollars (Mexican*) a reasonable fee for them?" I asked, seizing the moment to increase future hospital revenues.

"Truly, very small!"

"The Honorable General understands that no one else receives the special eye examination," I said, without blinking an eyelash. "That is for rare cases only."

Graciously he assured me that his body already felt better than in months, and he believed this was due primarily to the drops in his eyes. He would depend on me in the future to help keep him and his staff in good condition.

When he had gone I sank weakly into a chair, struggling to puzzle out the reason for his visit. It was possible, of course, that he did feel better, although my treatment had certainly done nothing toward that end. Even if it had, there was no need for him to make a

---

* A Mexican dollar was then equal to about forty cents in gold.

personal call at my home. Slowly my admiration grew for this official who, with every power at his command and with pride as his strongest racial trait, had nevertheless been sufficiently great-minded to explain to a young foreigner about a moment of weakness.

Perhaps the inescapable question of "face" was the chief factor here. It might be that having forfeited even one man's respect, the General had to set the matter right to his own satisfaction. Whatever the motivation, the act itself had its own virtue. Politician with a dubious past he might be, but I could not keep from wondering how many Westerners in like circumstances would have done as much to smooth an unpleasant situation. In that hour Chinese stock went up several points, forcing me to admit that my original mental set about these people was about to be subjected to radical changes.

Nephritis was a minor ailment with General Chang; the real trouble was syphilitic, temporarily in a state of remission. He reacted most favorably to proper treatment, and almost overnight the American hospital received some widespread publicity. Chungking papers carried headlines to the effect that its foreign doctor, by dropping a little medicine in an important official's eyes and injecting a needle or two in his arm, had cured him of a complication of serious diseases. What was considered even more remarkable was that no treatment was forced on a patient that the physician would not first submit to himself. It promptly became the fad for Chungking leaders to seek us out and, while I personally felt ever more asinine among my medical colleagues, this absurd advertising led to a decided increase in hospital prestige and earnings. Also it proved the truth of the Chinese saying: "To become a famous doctor, a man needs only a little learning."

More important from the personal angle was the friendship that resulted with a Chinese business man named Lin. Even in our first professional meeting, I found myself attracted to this patient. At that time Lin was in the prime of life, about forty-four years old; like most Szechuenese he was well-built, with clean-cut features and an unusually open countenance. When I discovered that he spoke English fluently, my satisfaction knew no bounds. Examination proved him to be the victim of chronic nephritis, a case far in advance of the General's and complicated by high blood pressure. This second condition is rarely found among Chinese, and its absence is due, I believe, to the leisurely tempo of normal Chinese life. In reply to intelligent questioning, I told Lin exactly what was the matter and outlined the specific dietary regimen and medication essential to recovery.

On his return for a second appointment it was clear that he had read everything available in Chungking on kidney diseases. This information, added to the smattering of Western science he had acquired as a youth in an American college, provoked all sorts of discussions. I began to look forward eagerly to his visits. In this instance there was no interpreter as a barrier between two minds, and our conversations soon ranged from medicine to local politics, taxation, finance, and world affairs. In each of these fields of thought my new acquaintance displayed an intellectual grasp that kept me, the Westerner and younger man, on my toes mentally.

Our growing friendship, however, was not to be all "beer and skittles," for through it I was to come, for the first time, face to face with the original Great Wall of China. This, built of family law and filial tradition, rather than the stone and mortar used by Chin-hsi Hwang-ti in the third century B.C., was even more effective in keeping out foreign "barbarians" and their innovations than was the "First Emperor's" magnificent feat of engineering. For Lin, despite intelligent response, did not improve as he should have done. When confronted with my demand for truth, he murmured regretfully that his household, considering the diet regulations absurd, refused to prepare the prescribed foods.

"Have you no say in the matter?" I asked, nettled by such an excuse.

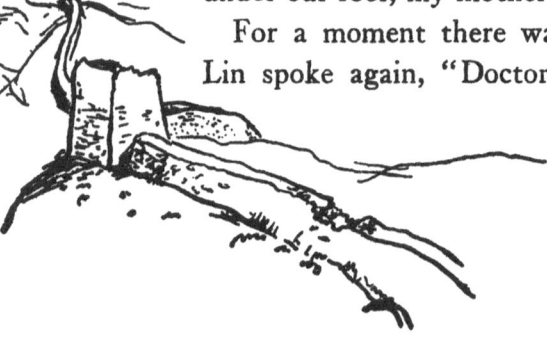

"Of a certainty! But when I scolded the women under our roof, my mother wept."

For a moment there was silence between us, then Lin spoke again, "Doctor, you are a foreigner who has been here too short a time to become acquainted with Chinese customs. My parents, believing our ancestors' ways the right ones, think that this strange diet will only harm me in the end. Moreover, when a woman makes up her mind," he shrugged his shoulders in a gesture of tolerant finality, *"mi teh fa!"*

I could not control a brief frown over the use of this Chungking *Tu Hwa* (Earth Language), expression, *mi teh fa*. A vulgarism of the Mandarin *muh iu fa tz*, meaning "there is no other way," it was becoming all too familiar to my ears, since it was used to settle any and every argument. "Then your parents would never agree to your coming into the hospital, would they?" I asked slowly.

Lin was thoughtful. "It may be I can arrange to do so. Still, you must know, Doctor, that they will bring me food on each visit."

"Yes, but like all other patients, you will eat nothing while they are present, and after they leave, your nurse will take care of such gifts."

I never learned what arguments were used to accomplish our ends, but within a few days I had Lin safely under my supervision in the hospital. There, as expected, none of the callers came empty-handed. Steaming containers of sweetened eggs, or pork richly browned in sauces, so heightened by Szechuen condiments that even a taste left the mouth burning, appeared one after the other and one after the other was confiscated. Almost at once he began to show definite gain, and I to add several ounces to my bony frame. Maud, unaware of the tempting delicacies I was sampling in the hospital, found it difficult to reconcile my improved physical appearance with an apparent loss of appetite at meals.

"I feel like a different man, my friend," the patient told me when he had been there for about three weeks. "Would that I might remain here for another month!"

"Another month at least!" I insisted confidently, despite the question raised by this remark. "By the time you go home, you will be so much better that your people will understand and help you." I could not refrain from adding, "You certainly have good cooks at your house." For a second the patient seemed puzzled, then as understanding came, he laughed heartily.

"Doctor," he told me one morning, "I must leave tomorrow. My parents know only unhappiness that I prefer to remain here rather than under our own roof, and at their honorable age I dare not cause them to squeeze heart—better it is that I myself be ill."

That anyone, so well versed in modern science and so highly intelligent in every other respect, could make such a statement floored me. For the moment I longed to voice bitterly my sense of frustration against these filial laws that hung a strangling noose about present-day China's neck, but I managed to hold my tongue.

Lin had been brought up on a code strangely resembling the Gloria's theme: "As it was in the beginning, is now, and ever shall be," and neither maturity nor foreign influence was sufficiently strong to release him from the submission such training demanded.

When the patient left, he exacted my promise to attend a feast at his home one day in the following week. This, an elaborate affair, proved most enjoyable and was succeeded by other numerous evidences of his kindness. As time went on, Lin continued to keep professional appointments regularly, and to my deep satisfaction seemed to be sustaining the level of his hospital improvement.

Meanwhile, I was serving more hours daily in the *ih yuen* (healing hall), the Chinese term for hospital, and having increasingly close contacts with the Chung-kingese as patients and as fellow-citizens. During the Period of Great Heat, now upon us, the city resembled an overheated oven, but my background of humid Maryland summers made adaptation to this trying climate fairly easy. High temperature seemed to have little effect on the living habits of the Chungkingese. They resorted to few Western methods of keeping cool and continued, as far as I could discover, to eat and drink food as hot as that consumed in midwinter.

On the streets at every possible opportunity now I could not forbear staring when a customer, throwing down a copper cash on a food-vendor's counter, caught up one of the popular fried-bread-twists still smoking hot with grease, and stuffed it into his mouth. Even my fingers, toughened by sterilizing processes, could not have handled the object without discomfort, and I never ceased to wonder how the more sensitive surfaces of the tongue and palate could endure such heat. This ability could not be attributed to habitual performance, since young children showed much the same degree of facility as adults, and Lamarck's theory of acquired characteristics seems more plausible here than in many other instances. Perhaps generations of consuming hot food and drink have dulled the tissue sensitivity of lips, tongue, and larynx.

While most articles of food were exposed not only to all the germs that flourished in Chungking's filth-weighted atmosphere but to flies and handling as well, two delicacies, at least, were given a primitive sort of protection. The roasted fowls hanging temptingly from food-shop ceilings wore a rich coat of red brown shellac; eggs were kept edible for months, and even years, by being embalmed in a cement made from lime, clay, and rice chaff.

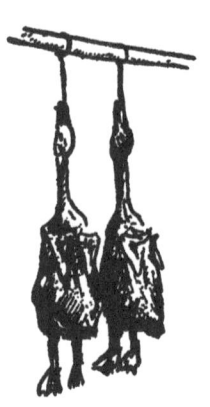

As my knowledge of these people increased, I decided that two of their greatest assets toward longevity were deliberation and a highly developed sense of humor. Regardless of his individual importance in commercial or official world, a Chinese can almost always find time to *sua ih ha tz*, another Tu Hwa expression which means "to play a little." Sitting with a companion or two at a small, square table in one of the city's innumerable tea-houses, he loses himself completely in pleasant conversation over a bowl of freshly brewed leaves. In these odd moments of social exchange men know complete relaxation such as Westerners rarely experience in the course of a day.

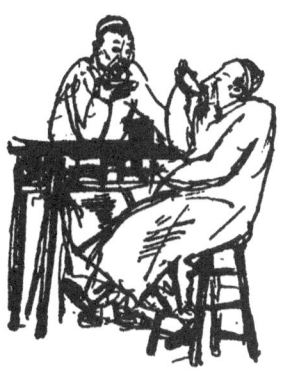

Later, when I also had acquired the custom of dropping into China's "hot-soda-fountains" for a drink of tea, I found myself envying the ability of my companions to cast care and responsibility aside. Even while laughing and talking, I, typically American in mind-processes, was restlessly conscious of some patient's failure to improve, or the amount of research I needed to do in order to become of greater use in this field. In sharp contrast to our own ways, there, where life for the average citizen was a desperately difficult ordeal, self-preservation had taught the individual to squeeze the utmost in enjoyment from every possible moment. Some foreigners chose to call this quality in the Chinese laziness—an absurd criticism of a race that works much longer hours and for much less reward than does the average American or European.

My habit of visiting tea-houses first began as a matter of professional policy. The breach between foreign physician and Chinese patient seemed unnecessarily wide to me. It was caused, I believe, not only

5

by alien backgrounds but by the inequalities of a situation in which the foreigner was usually at his best and the native at his worst. Relaxing in the teahouses, men met on more even grounds, drank their refreshing bowls of tea, and exchanged ideas on every conceivable subject. China is the most democratic nation on earth and, except when topics verged on the scholastic, the coolies present were just as likely as merchants or scholars to join in the general discussions.

As my Chinese vocabulary enlarged, these free-for-all arguments became increasingly enjoyable and, whenever opportunity offered, I slipped in a word about modern medicine and the hospital's value to the community. Through this medium the institution received interest and patronage from many people who might otherwise never have given it a moment's consideration.

My own gains were immeasurable, for these social contacts with the Chungkingese were entirely natural, revealing racial traits usually kept under cover in the sober dignity of hospital rooms. Among these a sense of humor was paramount. Everything is grist for the Chinese mills of laughter, and that I might contribute in person to this amusement supply I discovered with dismay, one hot afternoon in late August.

Bound for a social affair in the first range of Hills, I started out attired in the best white linen suit and the only London cravat my wardrobe afforded. As was my custom when using a chair, I had tucked a book under my arm. On this day the volume, bound in rich red cloth, was Osler's *Medicine*. As soon as my coolies swung into the business section, I became aware that something out of the ordinary was afoot.

Most unusual for Szechuen where moisture is usually plentiful, this particular year the rainy season was long overdue. The land lay scorched, and crops, maturing too fast in the pitiless heat, had turned sere and yellow. Farmers were afraid to sell their small stores of food, and prices in the city had begun to soar. As a result, the Chungkingese, co-operating with the countryside, had decided to stage an ancient ceremony of praying for rain.

At first glance the performance seemed somewhat like a visiting Fireman's Convention at home, with an endless parade winding up and down the streets of stairs, attended by a generous quota of noise. Citizens dressed in their best vied for attention with the bizarre paper dragons and similar monsters that were a large part of the procession. Everywhere along the line of march, columns of smoke rose from small burning piles of idol paper and sticks of incense.

The officiating priests and acolytes were costumed as ferocious animals or demons from the spirit world. Over their faces these wore masks sufficiently hideous to scare the wits out of anyone even in broad daylight. To their headgear, square or oblong in shape, were appended long red streamers or, in some cases, what

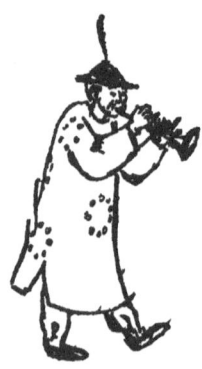

looked to me like bamboo sprouts with six or eight lighted sticks of incense radiating from the center of these. Each group of priests was preceded by dancers and musicians, playing instruments, exploding fire-cracker strings, or merely yelling. One man, dressed in robes of tarnished gaudiness and a veiled hat, carried a long sword, which he swung continuously in a curving stroke from one side of the narrow street to the other.

At periodic intervals coolies on the curbs flung buckets of muddy Yangtze water directly in the path of the paraders, forcing them to jump nimbly out of the way to avoid a wetting. The coolies' aim proved, in many instances, only too accurate, and the bedraggled victims, conscious of providing that touch of hilarity which Chinese seem to enjoy even at the most serious moments, joined good-naturedly in the amusement at their expense. Completely fascinated by so interesting an exhibition, I forgot as we moved along with the crowd that a foreigner might offer special attraction as target. When a bucketful finally hit me, the surprised indignation on my face must have been amusing in the extreme, for the spectators roared.

In a split second gay cravat and red book lent streams of color to my sopping suit, and I gave instant voice to an ejaculation which my training in tender years had warned me was never used by "nice people." Unfamiliar as these Chungking citizens were with English, they understood this epithet without difficulty and shouted anew. For a moment, ruined in appearance and physically uncomfortable, I glared at all about me, but in the face of their enjoyment, my ill-humor faded and I, too, grinned. At once I had a sudden, indescribable feeling of being accepted in this strange world. After that, it seemed a trivial matter to return home and change before proceeding to my destination.

Old China hands have an unfailing supply of tales concerning the value of humor in solving Chinese problems, serious or otherwise. Frequently, this quality shared in common provides a basis for friendship and oils the machinery of business. On a number of historic occasions foreigners in China have actually saved not only their property but their necks by a fortunate quip or jest. Perhaps the feeling about "face" makes the Oriental dread ridicule beyond most torments, and, accordingly, the Chinese consider it important for a man to accept gracefully those tricks of fortune that make him the object of other men's amusement.

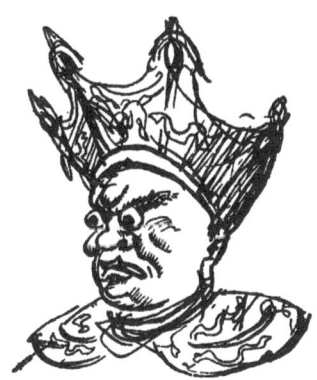

CHAPTER V

A Wandering Kite with a Long, Long Tail

Most convincing to Chinese faith in traditional ceremonies was the fact that rain, weeks overdue, now fell within twenty-four hours. Making up for lost time, each day strove to outdo the former in illustrating their expressive phrase, "sky emptying buckets." The first of September we moved back from the Hills to the city, hoping to elude the greater mold and moisture of those shaded slopes at the risk of higher temperature. Chungking continued to steam, and the cracks in flagstone streets became fissures through which oozed the dank filth of ages. The Chungkingese philosophically accepted their trying atmosphere, but most foreigners were mentally and physically the worse for wear, excepting those who had been fortunate enough to summer on distant O Mei Hsan, where an altitude of eleven thousand feet added to the attractions of a sacred mountain.

The newcomer in the Orient is always shocked by free discussion among foreigners of subjects usually under taboo in polite society at home. Some of this is due, undoubtedly, to the fact that the Chinese never fails to call a spade "a spade." To him the body's normal physical processes are perfectly natural, and he sees no reason for not mentioning these as freely as any other subject. While traditional ritual of virtue has made the Chinese woman more circumspect than most about covering her body in public, she, like her husband, considers foreign squeamishness artificial.

It is the Anglo-Saxon whose sensibilities are most easily shocked, for the Continental European is nearly as frank in such matters as the Oriental. But, after a few months of living where an elderly Chinese may, without loss of dignity, use a roadside ditch for an emergency evacuation; or where, in all courtesy he may ask your wife if and when she expects to have a child, it seems rather useless to cling rigidly to one's own code.

The prevalence of intestinal infections contributes another influential factor. In a climate like that of Chungking, where almost no foreigner escapes diarrhea or dysentery in some form, such ailments become common topics of conversation socially.

The very seriousness of such diseases challenges the victims to treat them lightly. When a man knows that his intestinal trouble is quite likely to ruin his career on the field and ship him home to a life of semi-invalidism, he considers it good sportsmanship to discount the threat, at least in conversation with others. It took no small courage to fight the losing battle with climate and disease as valiantly as did many of the foreigners in Chungking. Usually it was a losing one; if they had doubts of this, the foreign cemetery and the lengthy list of workers at home on furlough soon corrected optimism.

In October, one of our friends, who was skipper of a Yangtze Rapids steamer, called on arrival in port and brought an invitation for Maud to spend a month in Ichang with his wife. Maud had stood her first Chungking summer badly, and since Ichang's present temperature was less enervating than ours, I overcame her objections to the proposal and insisted on her acceptance.

One morning Doctor Strobel, to whom I was turning more often than to anyone else in Chungking's medical world, stopped at the hospital. "I hear you're about to travel," he began.

"Not I! Maud went down to Ichang last week, if that's what you mean."

"No, you're going into Southwest China on an important case."

"Well, it's news to me."

He smiled. "The Chinese know all about it, if you don't. I wanted to give you a word of advice. If you go, make certain your contract for fees and expenses is clearly understood before taking a step. In this instance you'll be dealing with politicians, not with Chinese business men."

For several hours following his call, I went about wondering if all Chungking were to be informed before me. But in the late afternoon, I was told that a committee from the Provincial Governor was awaiting me in the hall. Since I could still speak only the simplest Chinese phrases, I called as usual on Doctor Tu, as interpreter. One of the heads of the Central Government at Nanking on an official trip to the Southwest had, it seemed, become ill and needed immediate attention. At that time, there were no aerial routes to the Southwest, and Chungking, several hundred miles distant as the crow flies from where he was staying, was the nearest point at which modern medical attention might be procured.

Born though I was with an itching foot, for the first time in life a journey made no appeal. Time and thought these days were fully occupied with routine work and plans for hospital reorganization.

"This great honor is deeply appreciated," I had Tu tell their spokesman, "but I cannot accept."

The Chinese merely considered this refusal the correct opening response and continued to discuss the proposition in detail.

They offered to supply an interpreter, a bodyguard of soldiers, all expenses, and twenty-five dollars (Mexican) a day for services. The phrase, "all expenses and twenty-five dollars a day," caught my attention. Six months in Chungking had taught me that the first

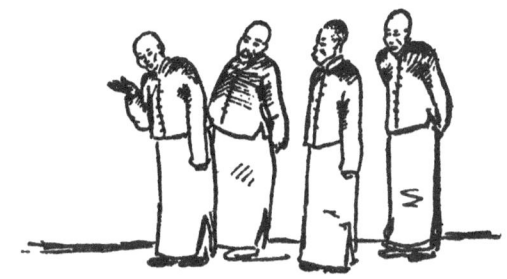

sum mentioned in a bargain was always but a fraction of the amount finally paid. The hospital needed ready money badly, and this might be a good way to earn some, provided I could find freedom to go. "Tell them," I urged Tu, "that the trip is worth five hundred dollars a day." This ridiculous figure encouraged the committee to get down to business.

No Oriental ever agrees to the original offer on anything; to do so would place him at once in the category of *tai lao* (too credulous and honest to be good for anything—a Chinese equivalent for "sucker"). Had I been sufficiently interested to consider their first proposal, the Committee would probably have found a courteous excuse for seeking medical help in other quarters.

Though the prospective patient was, by hearsay, enormously wealthy, I had no personal desire to gouge either the government or its representative in this case. It seemed only fair, however, that the hospital should gain something from an arrangement that necessitated a long, dangerous journey for a physician who had plenty to do at home, and that exposed to possible damage or loss the numerous expensive instruments and drugs which would have to be carried as equipment. In Chungking, one does not call up the wholesale house and order new surgical appliances delivered at once, even if money be available—as it usually was not. Should you break the only electric cautery the staff possesses, you might, with good luck, get another in a month or two from Shanghai, or in three or four months from America.

With these complications in mind, I began to bargain in true Oriental fashion and ignored all offers until the figure had climbed to one hundred fifty. Then I spoke. "For two hundred dollars a day (Mexican) I agree to go. It is not my wish to make this journey, and I do so only as a special favor to His Excellency, the Governor of Szechuen. In return I wish his seal on our contract as well as on travel permits all along the way." This was following Strobel's advice to secure local backing; with the Central Government more than a thousand miles distant at Nanking, it became highly important that Szechuen's powerful warlord stand behind this enterprise.

"When can *Beh Ih-seng* leave?" was the immediate response to my two-hundred-dollar ultimatum.

"At once! The patient will have long enough to wait as it is."

Promising to make all travel arrangements, provincial visés, and financial contracts ready by the next dawn, the committee left.

I was in the pharmacy sorting out drugs and laboratory chemicals to take along, when my friend, Lin, arrived. China has an amazing grapevine system of news-spreading and he, like Strobel, was already conversant with every detail of the proposed trip.

"So now you select drugs," he commented with a smile.

"Yes, and no matter which ones I take they will probably be wrong. I haven't an idea what's troubling the patient."

"For my country's sake, I ask you to choose well— he is a valuable man."

I chuckled. "Wonders will never cease! A Szechuenese actually speaking in favor of a Nanking official."

Lin's eyes twinkled, then he changed the subject: "Would you like one or two of my men to accompany you and smooth the way? The journey will be through a very wild section of our land. Also, it will be beautiful—almost I envy you. Once my father traveled down the old Mandarin Road. He has never ceased telling us of the scenery. Your way does not lead to Burma, but the ranges are equally magnificent, it is said."

"I wish you were coming along," I told him, "but I see no need for your men. The committee has promised to provide interpreter and bodyguard, and I shall take Lao-mi from the hospital as personal servant."

"Did they advise you about clothing?"

"Clothing? No, why should they?"

"Truly, you are young, and a *t'sai-lai-tih* (newcomer)," Lin mocked, "or you'd know the reputation of those mountains. But lay down your heart! I will see that you do not freeze to death." He rose to go. "Take good care of yourself, Doctor."

I squinted at a bottle in my hand. "Will you do as much?"

"Of a certainty!" he promised lightly and left.

A little later, Lin's servant appeared with a package. This contained two complete winter outfits, rich blue and gray satins lined with soft white fur. As I packed them into my bag, an apparently absurd procedure this November afternoon in Chungking at 80° Fahrenheit, I thought anew of their owner and wondered anxiously if his family were again refusing to co-operate.

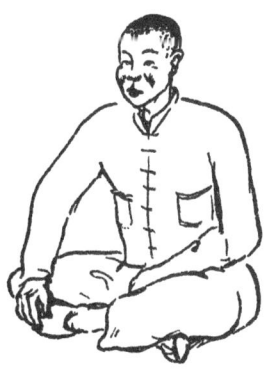

By six o'clock next morning, as planned, I was ready to leave, but except for Lao-mi and a hospital coolie who would accompany us to the water's edge, I seemed singularly alone in this purpose. Two hours later the interpreter arrived and at nine, my sixteen chair-coolies —four shifts to share the strain of carrying in high altitudes. To these were added shortly before noon the ten soldiers that composed the bodyguard. Suddenly, like characters in their own Shadow Shows, one after the other of these worthies disappeared from the scene, leaving me again entirely alone, "all dressed up and no place to go." Gradually each returned from his particular errand or excursion, and at four o'clock when the committee chairman, who had promised to get us through the Chungking City Gate to the river, at last joined us, we actually set out.

At the water-gate, where customs guards examined papers and baggage, all went "merry as a marriage

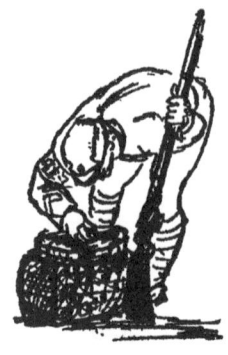

bell" until I saw them lift the lid of the *mei hsiang tz* (covered wicker basket lined with oiled paper) in which I had placed medical equipment.

"Tell them not to touch that!" I shouted to the interpreter. "Everything in there has been sterilized." I had personally seen to this and to placing the instruments cotton-wrapped for immediate use in oiled-silk bags, since it was unlikely I'd find facilities for doing so where I was going. For several moments my go-between protested, explaining that these tools to heal a high official of the Central Government must not be handled, but his efforts were to no avail.

"The National Government is undoubtedly the highest authority," he was informed, "but Chungking is Chungking, and its customs duties are our own affair and nobody else's. How do we know what you wish to smuggle into Kweichow?" finished the inspector belligerently, and once more lifted the lids.

I swung out of my chair and the next moment, to everyone's great surprise, I had replaced the lid and seated myself on top. This action, while protecting the instruments, was hardly conducive to progress, for the examiners and I, facing each other in that ancient city gate, presented the age-old problem of two immovable obstacles. Finally the distracted chairman received the assurance that a note from the Governor about this particular basket would give it exemption, and he hurried off to get it.

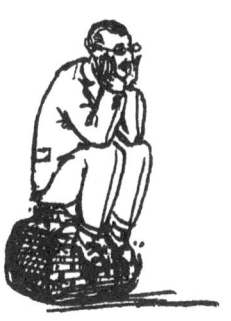

By the time the new document had been procured and accepted, dusk was turning the sky gray. Load-bearers once more adjusted baskets to carrying-poles, and the committee chairman came to bid me farewell and to repeat the names of the towns at which I would collect fees and expenses along the way.

"The money for today, what of that?" I asked.

"But *Beh Ih-seng* is just starting the journey," protested the chairman.

"Oh, no," I contradicted through the interpreter, "I have been traveling since six o'clock this morning, and it's been a long day, indeed."

"True," he agreed grudgingly. "Honorable Doctor, permit me to give you a note for payment of today's money when you return, so you need not carry that extra burden of silver on the road."

Strobel's warning concerning politicians reminded me that "a bird in the hand is worth two in the bush." "No burden at all," I assured him. "This servant who is returning to the hospital will gladly carry the money there for me."

When the chairman still hesitated, I added, "Perhaps I have misunderstood the Governor's terms of contract. Shall we return to find out?" Immediately the money was paid, and the servant departed with it.

Slowly we filed out the gate and down the steps to the river bank. With the evening meal now in preparation, this was a rare opportunity to get intimate glimpses of the community living outside the city wall. Here, against high mud banks, in an area which one might have supposed large enough to accommodate several dozens of people, dwelt as many thousands. Too desperately poor to afford the safety of living within the wall, these denizens of the water-front built their houses in ascending tiers against the rocky cliff. The foundations, bamboo poles, were secured simply by tying those of each level to the ones just below; and squares of matting on a flimsy framework made the roofs and walls.

Perpendicular ladders answered for common stairways to these ramshackle, one-room homes in which whole families existed, eating when there was food; toiling at every possible odd job; sleeping to dream, perhaps, of a rice bowl that was always filled.

Nourishment for this horde came chiefly from the Yangtze, their only ally in the precarious struggle to live, for the uncertain current offered a constant hazard to overloaded cargo boats poling down from the farmlands. Boatmen, trying to recapture purple eggplants or leafy green cabbages that had been jolted overboard, knew little success in competition with the fast-swimming water-front boys, whose trained sight could discover a floating prize almost before the original owner missed it.

Annually in late winter, the Yangtze, gorged by melting snow and ice from the Himalayan peaks that

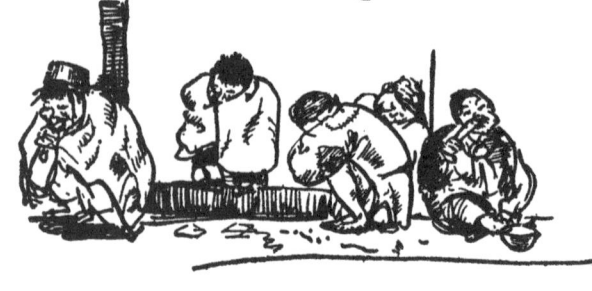

had given it birth, rose suddenly before Chungking to
a height ranging from thirty to ninety feet and demanded entrance. For a night, horror would reign outside the city wall. Under the impact of flood waters,
bamboo and matting huts snapped like matchsticks,
and many of the occupants, groping toward the heights
in darkness to the terrifying roar of angry waters, lost
footing and were seen no more. There were always
plenty of these unfortunates to take the place of the
missing and to begin promptly the task of rebuilding,
utilizing every scrap of debris in the process.

This evening, the glimmer of candle flame and the
red glow of charcoal beneath cooking pots lent these
huts a picturesque tone never to be seen in broad
daylight. Laughter punctuated the medley of chatter
and, strangely enough, the sinister quality commonly
associated with slums of the world was missing. As
we ferried across the river, I found myself puzzling
again over Chinese ability to endure the utmost in
misery and still not succumb.

By the time we reached the other shore, it was
already dark, but our procession, with numerous small
lanterns casting eerie shadows over the terraced fields,
swung along the narrow flagstone path that for centuries had led into Kweichow Province and on to the
great Southwest.

All during the summer this first and second range
of hills opposite Chungking had been alive with moving

6

bands of soldiers engaged in some minor, interprovincial conflict. Our *fu-to* (head of chair-coolies and load-bearers) now paused at every small settlement to make inquiries about the safety of continuing this night journey. At the first large village hè decided we were too close to the trouble zone to go on, so we stopped. The only inhabitant in sight was a sleepy gateman, and I began to wonder about accommodations.

"There is an inn, *Beh Ih-seng*," Lao-mi told me, "but very dirty, it is said."

"Well, I certainly don't want to sit in this chair all night. Let's go see it!"

We picked our way through the darkness to a shadowy building and knocked on the entrance. A muffled answer was followed by the sound of shuffling footsteps, then the front opened and we stepped within. The room was almost as dark as the street, but gradually I made out the sleeping forms of other men and decided to take a chance among them.

The floor of this one-room inn was clay. Through the years spittle and filth had accumulated until the surface was as slippery as rubber, and for each two steps forward I slid back one. This precarious footing, together with the single, wavering gleam of a bean-oil wick lost in a fog of opium smoke, gave the impression of a storm at sea; and for a second, I myself felt a little like the Ancient Mariner, alone in his company of traveling strangers.

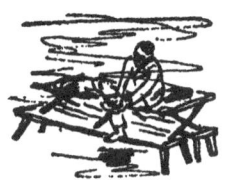

Lao-mi very efficiently discovered two empty wooden benches against one wall, and erecting my army cot on these, made up the bed. Removing shoes only, I climbed in between the covers and waited for supper. This, consisting of baked beans and a cup of prepared coffee, was swiftly consumed, and in spite of bad air and general unpleasantness, I fell asleep at once.

At three o'clock the *fu-to* roused us to start travel for the day. For breakfast tangerines were added to coffee and what remained of the first can of beans. The weather here was clear and much cooler than at Chungking and I walked for several hours, thereby pleasing my chair-carriers. We met soldiers everywhere along the way, and by mid-morning were halted and forbidden to go farther. The enemy, it seemed, lay just over this range, and if the day continued fair, a battle would undoubtedly occur in the afternoon.

While the *fu-to* and an officer harangued on the question of progress, I noticed that most of the rifles carried by these warriors had crooked barrels, and I asked the interpreter about them. In due time he explained that the men had shot off so many rounds of ammunition in practice the day before, that the barrels had melted and bent as a result. If the enemy followed the same policy, I thought there was little to fear from a battle. The decision, though, was to detour in a forty *li* (a li equals one-third mile) semicircle and avoid the battle line.

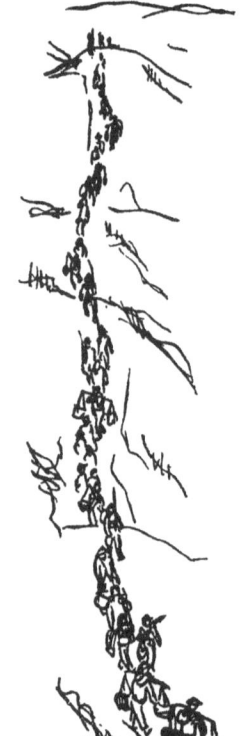

Reaching the walled town that marked the end of this additional journey, we were challenged by armed citizens who called themselves "Guardians of the Wall." On examination our papers proved to contain no mention of their township, and we were given the alternative of returning the way we had come or of submitting to a fresh customs assessment. While this latest discussion went on, I roamed about the gatehouse where an old woman sat beating cotton wadding to stuff her *pu-gai* (comfort) for the approaching winter.

The interpreter now came to whisper that the "Guardians" would waive the matter of customs if we would add several of their group to our bodyguard as a mark of good faith between us. This proposal smelt strangely like a "racket" to me, but weary of these numerous delays, I urged acceptance. The several turned out to be twenty, and we set off with these new recruits in our train.

That night was clear and sufficiently warm to permit our camping under the stars, a great improvement over my first experience with the inn. In packing, Lao-mi must have found a surplus of canned baked beans on the pantry shelves, for they continued to appear at every meal. Again I slept soundly until the three o'clock rousing signal.

Almost at once we began to climb, and the ascent lasted for several days. Progress slowed down enormously. I walked to save my coolies, and my first warning of rarefied air was the need to swallow constantly.

The party now halted frequently to rest, and on these occasions most of its members indulged in some form of opium, which, I learned after questioning, was considered an excellent "pick-me-up" in high altitudes. The drug's effect in rekindling energy was easy to understand, for it temporarily deadened the nervous system and distracted the mind from physical weariness and discomfort.

The surprising reaction was in blood pressure. Out of curiosity I tested a number of the men before and after taking the opium. The naturally high increase in pressure caused by thin air fell swiftly below normal, following each dose of the drug. I still have no theory to offer for this unusual performance.

On the second day of climbing, the men became exhausted at much shorter intervals, and I suggested larger food rations for all. To my amazement, Lao-mi served me eggs, canned bacon, and toast for lunch, three articles he had supposedly been keeping up his sleeve. We were now traveling on a narrow path cut from the cliff and strewn with fragments of rock—a constant menace to footing. Here, where one could look down for several thousand feet to a foaming river, a misstep would have meant certain death. Our party seemed to be in possession of these wild heights. No friendly villages appeared at regular distances as in the lowlands; instead, hours elapsed without our seeing a single hut.

In mid-afternoon we halted to eat where the path widened a little. As the meal came to an end, a band of soldiers appeared from around the bend, claimed that they were provincial militia stationed in the pass to prevent smuggling between Szechuen and Kweichow, and insisted on examining our baskets. I held what little breath I had left when, by a turn of good fortune, they overlooked the basket of medical supplies. Accordingly, I made only slight protest as they helped themselves to several other articles, among these my camera. They were an ugly-looking lot and, had necessity for fighting arisen, I doubt that my escort, less well-acclimated, would have stood a chance of winning. Ever since I have regretted the loss of that camera, for with it went all photographic record of this interesting journey.

A few *li* farther on, we came to a hut and were stopped again for the same purpose. These men proved to be the real militia; the previous ones had been bandits clad in stolen uniforms. They permitted us to go on after the most superficial examination, and with rare unselfishness I insisted that they accept two tins of baked beans from our supply, as a mark of appreciation.

Snow and ice now added to the dangers of the path. I was using one of Lin's fur-lined robes over my own clothing and was still uncomfortably cold. Most of the coolies wore their usual cotton suits and straw sandals

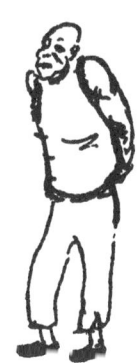

on bare feet. Only a few of the more fortunate among them had a sleeveless sheepskin jacket over the thin one, yet they made no complaints about the cold nor, as their meager supplies of opium gave out, about fatigue. Many of these Chungkingese had never seen snow, and they showed a childlike pleasure in handling it. "*Hao kan, hao kan!*" (Beautiful, beautiful!) they exclaimed repeatedly.

That night we stayed in a wayside rest-house, a crude shelter erected by some well-to-do Buddhist anxious to gain merit through good deeds. I bundled up in both of Lin's robes and was duly thankful for his thoughtfulness, for the cold was beyond description. This with the thin air made sleep almost impossible, and I rose the next morning feeling more weary than at bedtime.

It was soon apparent that the others felt the same way, for the men would push forward a few hundred feet and drop in their tracks. My own heart was thudding painfully, and bleeding noses left a sanguine trail behind us. As we circled around the peak, the foaming river again came into sight but was now so far below that we could identify it as water only where the rapids boiled white. In late afternoon the path began to descend, and by nine o'clock when a village was finally reached, we had begun to feel once more like normal human beings. As I recall it, this inn was worse than the previous one, but that night I was too jaded even to care.

The following evening we came to the town where I was to make my first collection of fees and expenses. Wondering about the safety of carrying so much money with me, on arrival I had Lao-mi inquire about missionaries, and learned that there was a small English Church Station in this place. The next move was to find the man who held the funds. After an exchange of courtesies, he began listing excuses for not handing over the sum due. Finally with patience gone, I had the interpreter warn him that unless the money were immediately forthcoming, I would turn back to Chungking next morning.

With the cash in hand, I made straight for the church compound and there saw the silver, exchanged for a Mission check on Shanghai, carefully deposited in a safe. This amount would be discounted a little down river, but the precaution would pay in the end, I felt sure. After this I soaked in a hot bath, changed garments, ate a meal that had no beans in it, and slept in a real bed.

CHAPTER VI

Solving a Chinese Puzzle

An hour out of town next morning we were halted
by a group of armed men in civilian clothes, who demanded the sum of money paid me the night before.
When my statements, plus the Mission check, finally
convinced them that their effort was fruitless, it was
suggested that I add five of their number to the bodyguard. I protested vigorously, but to no avail.

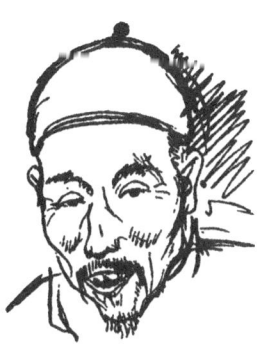

Lack of experience in China and my slight knowledge
of the language made me almost powerless on this journey. Under the circumstances, the interpreter and the
fu-to were the real managers, and I was forced to
accept their decisions. Gradually I began to suspect
the reasons for increasing the party on every possible
occasion. Here in this Chinese hinterland, as elsewhere
in the world, communities were eager to profit in every
way from tourists, particularly one supported by the
Government, and my coolie representative was doubtless offered "squeeze" to hire unemployed citizens.
Salary and food came from my expense account—a
matter to trouble nobody but the politicians and
me. I began to understand how almost any man with

ambition and a little money in China could acquire an army and, in time, become a warlord.

"How did those citizens know the amount I'd been paid?" I later asked the interpreter.

"In this district," he explained, "the Governor of Szechuen has few friends. However, he is a fierce general and when he asks favors, wise men grant them. Last night you were paid what you asked, *Beh Ih-seng*, but there was no good reason for not trying to get it back, was there?"

"And did they think I'd not have notified the Governor had the silver been taken from me?"

His eyelids hastily hid a flicker of amusement. "The town officials would have echoed your complaints with even stronger ones; they would have begged pity for having to live in a section overrun by bandits. And what could the Szechuen Governor say to that?"

Still descending the mountain, we made rapid progress. My chair-bearers had no difficulty carrying me now, so I rode once more. A surfeit of gorgeous scenery had given me esthetic indigestion, and I turned with satisfaction to a copy of Cabot's *Physical Diagnosis* and read for several hours. This day we did not halt for meals; everyone seemed to be devouring fruit, and I ate oranges, plentiful all over West China, until I lost count. I had supposed the unbroken march was to make up for lost time, but learned afterwards that the last foreigner to come along this route, a month or so

earlier, had been murdered, and my men were taking
no chances with their cargo.

The next day's landscape was reassuringly dotted
with settlements. I was startled by the fact that the
people hereabout neither looked nor acted like Chinese,
one outstanding physical difference being large and un-
shapely hands and feet. The interpreter explained that
they were Miaos, an aboriginal tribe, who had managed
to hold this Kweichow territory in spite of all Chinese
attempts during the centuries to oust them. They were
strong and sturdy-looking, but so unkempt and with
so little interest in things of the mind that the Chinese
had always scorned them as barbarians.

We found our halts in their villages amusing experiences. Many inhabitants, particularly children, had
never before seen a foreigner. After recovering from the
first astonishment, the more daring youngsters ventured closer to my chair, and when nothing dreadful
resulted from this, one or two stretched out fingers to
touch me. In return I offered them oranges, but instinct must have warned them against accepting gifts
from strangers, for the fruit was refused. Probably some
doubt existed in their minds and in those of their elders
about my exact classification among creatures, since my
Chinese companions and the tribespeople could not
speak each other's language.

We ate lunch in one of these villages. When Lao-mi
opened another of the inexhaustible cans of beans, then

heated and served me the contents, their excitement knew no bounds. I'd have given a good deal to be able to chart their thought processes about food that grew in tins. After this surprise, even the startling use of knife and fork was an anticlimax. Until that day I had always felt sympathy for exhibits in zoos and circuses. Now it seemed likely that all concerned shared in the diversion; certainly I enjoyed myself in this instance.

Soon the climbing began again. These particular mountains were sheltered from bitter winds, and the slopes were covered with bloom. Oddly enough I saw no animal life and no snakes, though these are common in the Chungking Hills. Of plants, *ma huang*, from which the drug, ephedrin, is derived, seemed most plentiful. The stems were covered with dark red berries, and my companions plucked and ate these as they marched. I tasted one or two but found them bitter.

By sundown we came to the town where I was to make another collection. When the business had been transacted and the money deposited at the resident Mission, I was attracted to a drugshop that had not yet closed its shuttered front for the night. On the shelves were jars containing snakes, frogs, and various insects in preservatives, and from walls and ceiling hung bunches of dried plant roots and stems. Showing the druggist the spray of *ma huang* I still carried, the interpreter questioned him about its curative qualities.

The old gentleman first explained carefully the theory to be found again and again in Chinese materia medica; namely, the importance of resemblance between parts of plant or animal producing medicines and the human parts affected by disease. For example, juice squeezed from the stems of *ma huang* is used to treat fevers, since fevers result from diseased blood conditions and blood flows through veins resembling stems. That taken from the joints of the plant is used, naturally, for arthritic joints and so on. Incidentally, this pharmacist had never heard of the drug's being applied locally as an astringent to mucous membranes—one of its commonest uses in the West. In China, whether given for fevers or for rheumatism, the chief reaction sought from it is profuse sweating.

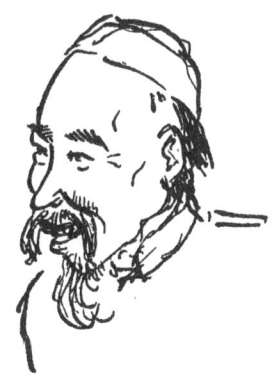

Again we were halted out of town next morning, then proving the money was safe elsewhere, once more added to the bodyguard. From this point the trail descended to a river bank, where company and baggage were loaded on a fleet of tiny boats. These narrow craft, pointed of bow and stern, had been specially designed to ride the rapids for which this waterway was famous, but they seemed extremely difficult to handle. While still close to shore one capsized and lost some of its baskets. Fortunately these contained nothing really essential to progress.

This trip, which lasted all day, was thrilling as well as beautiful. Approaching each of the rapids, the crews chanted weirdly in unison. The next moment we hurtled through space into a roaring, blinding maelstrom of seething water, only to emerge in a more placid stretch and there prepare for the succeeding plunge. Before the day was over, I felt sure that going over Niagara in a barrel was no trick at all, and I knew moments of thankfulness that Maud would hear nothing of these traveling details until too late to use her imagination.

In this wild, lonely country through which I had been journeying since Chungking, was some of Earth's most spectacular scenery. The Chinese are noted for making pilgrimages to beauty spots and will endure with little complaint all sorts of inconveniences along the way, but we had met almost no travelers. Civil strife and bandits apparently held the section in a paralyzing grip.

In amazing contrast, this same district today, less than ten years later, has become one of the most important sections for rehabilitating refugees. Here many thousands of them are engaged in a pioneering program of home-building and territorial development similar, in some respects, to that of our own West a century ago. In these secluded valleys persecuted civilians are safe, temporarily at least, from roaring guns and whistling bombs.

A modern motor road—in itself a superhuman achievement—now links the district with the other western provinces, and through these to Indo-China and

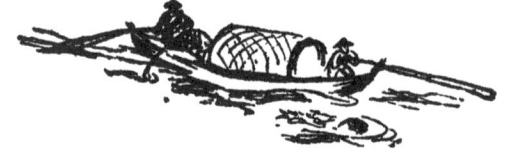

Burma. Over this highway winds a steady stream of homeless men, women, and children, their footsteps crowded by rickshaws, wheelbarrows, donkeys, and motor trucks carrying personal and government supplies of food and equipment. But when I saw it, all was just as it had been for hundreds of years.

Disembarking at a market town, I found that another day's journey across country would take us to our destination. There, resembling a kite with a long, overweighted tail, I finally arrived, accompanied by one hundred twenty bodyguards, *fu-to*, interpreter, personal servant, chair-coolies, and load-bearers. The size of my retinue must have made quite an impression on the guardians of Kweiting City, for they were most courteous. I learned that the patient I was seeking had reached this spot only an hour or two earlier, had stopped just long enough to talk with the Mayor and had then hurriedly taken the road to the West.

There was nothing to do but trail him, and to my surprise we caught up with his party a few *li* beyond in the farmlands. They were apparently expecting us—more grapevine—I suppose, and had made temporary camp. The sick man, a highly civilized product of excellent Chinese background and broad European education, was suffering from a bad carbuncle. This had been lanced, but not properly excised, and inflammation covered a large area. He agreed readily to my suggestion for operating at once; his ready confidence

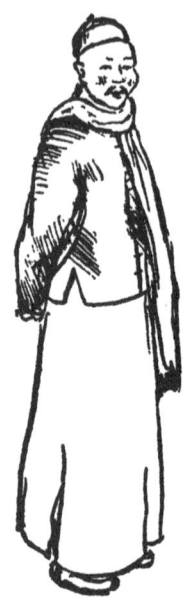

in me was undoubtedly inspired by the luxuriant goatee I had acquired from no shaving on the trip.

My second request—that we camp right here until the next day—did not meet with such favorable response. After weighing the matter carefully, he agreed to do so, provided I send my large party on ahead. "I, too, am on my way to Chungking, Doctor, so we can travel together," he assured me, "and these others will save time and silver by returning at once."

This arrangement was entirely satisfactory to me, and after I had selected Lao-mi, a load-coolie or so, and two shifts of chair-bearers, I sent the *fu-to*, interpreter, and others along with my blessing.

Later that afternoon when the operation had been performed and the patient was resting comfortably, I fished out laboratory chemicals from the jealously guarded *mei hsiang tz* and made blood and urine tests. These were anything but encouraging. Next morning while dressing the wound, I asked the patient if he couldn't find time to remain in the Chungking Hospital for a week or two.

"At present, there seems no reason why I should not," he assured me.

Each day of the return trip, on a route west of the one I had traveled to find him, it became clearer that this official's moves were shrouded with secrecy. To begin, his entourage was absurdly small for an important political figure. He avoided towns wherever

possible, frequently detouring through paddy-fields to
do so. Whenever altitude or weather forced us to seek
shelter for the night, it was usually in some small ham-
let so far from the beaten track that the word "Government" still meant Peking with the old Empress
Dowager on the throne.

Across the border in Szechuen we ran again into battle lines. Few of those soldiers carried rifles, bent or
straight; instead, their equipment seemed to consist of
knives or swords and umbrellas. Had the season been
warmer, fans also would have been in evidence. The
opposing factions were apparently on the best of terms,
except when battles were staged, for we saw them eating and gambling together in several villages. They did
nothing to delay us, and that seemed fortunate, since,
in spite of physical discomfort, my patient insisted on
advancing at top speed.

I attended to the dressing first thing each morning,
and while doing this on the day of expected arrival in
Chungking, he astonished me by saying quietly, "Since
our ways part shortly, Doctor, will you please give me
directions for further treatment?"

"But I'll take care of you myself while you're in the
hospital, and by the time you leave, this will probably
have healed."

His lips shaped a fleeting smile, but he eyed me
gravely. "My plans have been changed and I do not
go to Chungking—*muh iu fa tz'*"

7

I frowned. With the field of operation still draining, his condition warranted no risks. On second thought I realized that in this situation the patient, not the physician, would make the decision, and further argument seemed useless. When I finished, he expressed appreciation with the graciousness typical of his race, and made out a check much larger than the fee originally stipulated. Then satisfying himself that my men knew the direct route to Chungking, he bade me farewell and waved us out of sight. My last glimpse was of his standing in that Szechuen field in which we had eaten breakfast. Where he intended to go from there he had permitted none of us to know.

That afternoon when I entered the hospital office, Doctor Tu greeted me, added a compliment about my beard, then asked, "Where did you leave your patient, *Beh Ih-seng?*"

After answering in detail, I admitted that I was curious about the official's present whereabouts.

Tu led me to a window. "See that Government gunboat anchored out there? That has been waiting for a week to carry him down river to Nanking."

"*Hsi chi deh hen!* (very strange!) Why do you suppose he'd travel overland when he might go in comfort by water?"

The Chinese doctor shrugged. "Who can say? Perhaps an order from Nanking, perhaps some whisper of danger waiting in Chungking. *Beh Ih-seng* need not be told that Szechuen is only six-tenths loyal to the Central Government, *hsi puh hsi?* (Yes, no?)"

Well, China wasn't the first country in history to be divided against itself, I thought silently, and these Szechuenese were an independent lot anyway. Many of the most disastrous civil wars through the centuries had started right in this province. I counted out the amounts due the hospital; watched Tu suck in his breath at the size of the fee; then went home to soak in a bath, eat, and sleep. The house into which we had moved on return from the Hills now seemed a comfortless barn without Maud in it. I had word that she would be arriving next day on the steamer from Ichang, and to add a piquant touch to our meeting, I forbore shaving my goatee.

From my standpoint as well as that of the hospital management, the trip had been successful. The last collection for expenses was still to be made, but by the time *fu-to,* interpreter, and coolies had all presented greatly augmented claims, this sum vanished into thin air. Even so, the institution gained financially, to say nothing of increased prestige. While I would have preferred to complete my job instead of leaving the patient as I had been compelled to do, this did not lessen my appreciation of a journey in country almost never visited by Westerners. The next morning's discovery that the Government gunboat had slipped down river in the night reassured me. I felt certain that my official had boarded it somewhere below Chungking and was now safely en route to the capital and medical attention.

Maud, unfortunately, was not so well satisfied by the affair as I. Enjoying a period of social gaiety and relaxation in Ichang, she received her first word of my proposed journey just after an Armistice Day service in the Scotch Mission Chapel. At the close, one of the men approached her with the question, "Did you get your wire from Chungking?"

"What wire?" she demanded, instantly certain that such a telegram could mean nothing less than injury or sudden death for me.

"Your husband wired that he is going down to the Southwest to look after some patient."

She breathed relief. Then a woman companion exclaimed in horrified tones, "Southwest? Oh, you poor thing!" shook her head compassionately and walked away.

In the next few minutes Maud was told the following:

1. That I had set out on a long, difficult journey unattended except by coolies. Since I was comparatively a newcomer in the country with almost no command of the language, there was no telling where I might end.

2. That my mission was so dangerous that the Government had given me a large bodyguard.

3. That the ranges I must cross were infested with bandits, and a bodyguard of soldiers, however large, would be no match for those desperadoes.

4. That the altitude and temperature of the mountains offered almost certain death to an inexperienced traveler.

5. That in the past decade not more than a dozen foreigners had taken this route, and that most of them had never been heard of since.

As is frequently the case with the person most concerned in such affairs, my wife did not see the telegram for about forty-eight hours, the office having declared a two-day holiday. When she did, it stated only the barest facts about my plans, for I had purposely worded it briefly to make her think it a matter of ordinary routine. I had no way of knowing that Ichang was a bit short on news at the moment and was prepared to dramatize the trip from start to finish.

"And there I was," Maud complained bitterly when we were once more together at home, "forced to sit and look pleasant for sixteen days until the next trip of the Yangtze Rapids steamer to Chungking." With feminine inconsequence, she shifted abruptly from the main argument to comment, "When I do finally see you, you're wearing that awful goatee, of all things!"

"There's no pleasing women," I retorted. "The Chinese admire my beard extravagantly."

Her eyebrows lifted. "Well, I don't!" Then she resumed, "You certainly put an end to my vacation."

"Since you couldn't possibly catch up with me, why didn't you go on having a good time while there was the chance?"

"Isn't that just like a man? Go on having a good time, indeed! Why you might have been murdered for weeks before I'd even have known I was a widow!"

Our houseboy appeared and interrupted this conversation by announcing that the curtains and draperies the mistress had wished cleaned during her absence were ready for inspection. My wife followed him from the room, and when she discovered that the cotton ones had been brushed and the heavy silk ones laundered, exactly contrary to orders, she temporarily forgot all other matters.

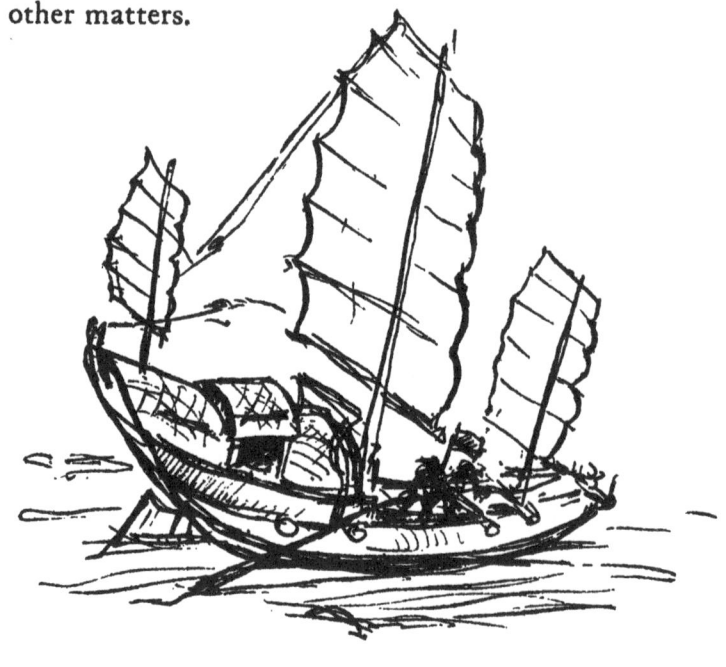

CHAPTER VII

Small Brother Lu

In China man's active day begins at dawn. The farmer goes to his field before the last stars have retreated from the sky. While the streets are still hushed with night, shop-front panels are lifted from their grooves, and the itinerant vendor's small charcoal fire pot casts the first warm glow of light upon a dusky world. Throughout Chinese history, rich and poor alike have been subject to this early-rising program. Officials were supposed to begin their duties on the same schedule as that used by the Imperial Government in Peking, where the ruler held his first conference with ministers around four in the morning.

Most foreigners tried to keep more nearly to Western working hours, but physicians were not among them, at least not in the interior. Pressure of medical work demanded a long day, and in Chungking with its intense heat and humidity the rule through a great part of the year, hospital operating rooms became infernos by mid-morning. Accordingly, Maud and I breakfasted most of the time at four or four-thirty, after which I went immediately to surgery. On arrival, I found the

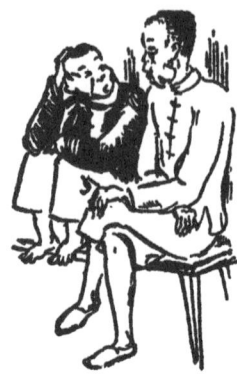

institution in active preparation for the day, with patients being fed and bathed and the building cleaned.

This early start cleared the decks for morning rounds, which had to be made between operating and dispensary hours. The clinics opened at nine and required the services of the two Chinese internes, twenty to twenty-five nurses, and me. Since this was a General Hospital treating men, women, and children, nurses belonged to both sexes. The dispensary was conducted as much like a modern American one as I could make it. To save time, drugs, dressings, and other routine necessities were arranged the night before in readiness for the long line of patients that waited for the doors to open.

Applicants moved, by turn, into an admission office, where a fee ranging from a few coppers to two dollars Mexican (charged according to financial ability and sometimes to the type of treatment needed), was paid and a receipt given. Those who could pay nothing were cared for from a special fund. At the next desk an attendant asked a simple question or two about the trouble, then gave out a numbered slip allocating the patient to the proper clinic: Medical, Surgical, Maternity, or Venereal, there to be examined and treated as turn came.

At the best the work in these clinics was hurried and superficial; thoroughness is an impossibility when hundreds of patients have to be cared for in two or three hours. I handled only the most puzzling and difficult cases, but no matter how fast I worked there was never sufficient time to study the condition as both training and personal interest demanded. Here, before my eyes, were all the rare diseases that I had dreamed of on first reading that travel pamphlet, and many more as well, for every conceivable malady and deformity came through that dispensary doorway. Yet, it was often hours later in the day that I realized with a flash some peculiar aspect of a case of which I had not been conscious when I was handling it in clinic.

Tuberculosis, syphilis, cancer, tumors, smallpox, muscular paralysis, beriberi, elephantiasis; fevers, dysentery, diarrhea, these three of every imaginable type; and abnormalities from a foot with four toes to the astonishing case of a Cyclops not only come to birth but to the teen-age.

In this last particular instance, an interne came to me as I cleansed and dressed an ulcer that had already eaten away most of a man's thigh and said, "*Beh Ih-seng*, I have a patient you may want to look at; before we have not seen or heard of anything like him."

A few minutes later I joined him and, unable to believe my own eyes, stared at the case in question. For a Szechuenese the youth was unusually small. His head had ears larger than average, but was otherwise normal in size and shape. It was the boy's face that evoked horror and pity. The mouth, revealing badly decayed front teeth, was tiny and round. Above it were two nostrils opening into a flat surface, where the nose's bony structure might naturally have been, and several inches above these, in the middle of what answered for a forehead, was one eye. His immediate trouble was a fulminating skin disease which was promptly treated. We plied him with questions about past history, but his intelligence quotient was too low for satisfactory answers. Later, inquiries on the street produced no responsible relatives, and his neighbors, apparently terrified by the youth's appearance, would not even discuss him.

Skin diseases were legion. Scabies were most common, though Hongkong Foot (similar to athlete's foot in the Occident) and leprosy ran as close seconds.

Aboard one of the United States gunboats, unexpectedly grounded by low water at Chungking, was a very pleasant young medical officer. Having had almost no practical experience and bored by idleness, he asked if he might attend clinic one morning. He came, as agreed, and while the rush was at its height, went from one section to the other observing. When I was free to give him some attention, he asked if I would show him a few of my own more interesting cases. "I am specially interested," he assured me, "in anything uncommon to Western medical practice."

I looked about for a moment, then found one that answered the requirements. "Put on a mask, then we'll take a look at this man," I suggested.

"My, he's a funny-looking patient," remarked "Navy," lifting up the sufferer's hand for closer examination. "I don't believe I've ever seen anything quite like this at home."

"No, you probably haven't," I replied, struggling to hide a flicker of humor. That the man had an odd appearance was true enough; he lacked hair, eyelashes, and fingernails, and his skin was as smooth and shiny as a billiard ball.

"This *must* be a rare case."

"Plenty of them out here."

"What do you call it?"

"Just plain leprosy."

"Leprosy, and you let me handle him!"

"Why not? With your breathing passages protected, there is no danger—none of his sores are suppurative."

He gave me a long look. "If I shove off now," he told me, without further comment about the case, "I'll just be able to reach the ship for tiffin." Then scrubbing up zealously, he left and I saw him no more.

While almost every other affliction known to man was common in Chungking, mental diseases were negligible in number. Chinese, as the saying goes, have their heads firmly screwed on their shoulders. The masses occupy body and mind completely in the business of food-getting, and among women, even the wealthiest, are kept so busy bearing children that neuroses rarely have a chance to develop. Syphilis is as

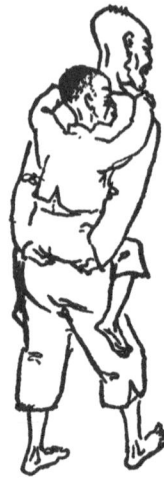

common as in America, but I cannot remember a single Chinese who had the brain complication that frequently accompanies that disease. When life becomes unendurable for a "Middle Kingdom" man, he seeks escape by suicide rather than by some other more complicated mental outlet.

Walking from the dispensary to the street, I noticed, many times over a period of several weeks, a small crippled boy who rode pickaback on a gnarled old coolie. Sometimes they were stationed close to our doorway; on other mornings the two would occupy a front-seat table at the small tea-house opposite our gate. Always the child eyed me intently from head to foot, and when he and the servant finally appeared in clinic one morning, I felt as if we were old acquaintances.

He was ten years old and his surname was Lu. Giving the case personal attention, I learned from the history card that the boy, due to a fall that had injured one leg in babyhood, had not walked since. The attendant added the information that having tried several native doctors without success, the youngster's family thought nothing more could be done for him. Since their son seemed certain to die before long, they permitted him freedom in all his ways and it was he, not they, who had chosen to try the foreigners as a last resort.

As his trousers and bandages were removed, I asked, "Do you live near by, *Lu Dih-dih* (Small Brother)? Many times I have seen you on our street."

"No, Honorable Doctor," he answered with a sharp glance, "I heard that sick people were carried into this Healing Hall and walked out well. This I wished to see for myself. It was true; therefore I am here."

The old servant now leaned over me anxiously as I began to examine the boy's leg. "Great Foreign Healer, you will not hurt him, *hsi puh hsi?* Already many doctors have done so."

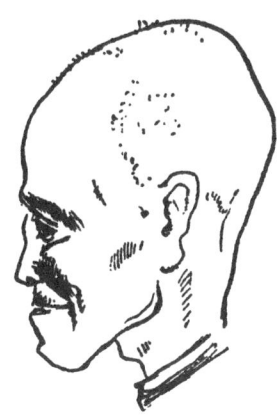

"Be quiet, Lao Er!" his young master commanded. "I do not fear."

"Truly, this patient is a man!" I exclaimed in Chinese, and saw the drawn, childish mouth shape into a grin.

He had little to grin about, I told myself, for his hip showed every sign of advanced bone tuberculosis, and on it were the scars of the treatments the coolie had mentioned. While he talked as an adult, his body was so small and emaciated that one could hardly believe he was ten years old.

"You say his parents did not come?" I inquired of my assistant. Then, "Do they have any money?"

"A little, so this servant tells me; enough to hire him and to pay these dispensary charges, perhaps."

"This is not a clinic case. He should go into the hospital for operations and months of treatment."

I turned again to the young patient. "*Hao puh hao* (good, not good) you come live in my hospital for a while? There we shall try to help your leg."

"You cannot do it today, Honorable Foreigner?"

"*Puh mang!* (Do not be in such a hurry!)" I told him, lifting my brows high at the very suggestion. "Eight years you have a bad leg, then in fifteen minutes you expect me to make it good—*ai-ya!*"

Fun lit his eyes once more. "For how long?"

"I do not know, Small Brother; perhaps several moons."

He sighed, as if weighing all that had gone before in his short life and this added prospect of new torment. "One question I would ask Foreign Healer: Will I then be able to walk?"

My mind risked the plunge. "I hope so."

He reached out and caught my hand. "It is your meaning, Honorable Doctor, that some day I may play like other boys?"

"It may be that some day you will play like other boys," I answered with gravity to equal his own.

"Then I will come," he promised firmly and continued half to himself, "Lu Dih-dih to walk and perhaps to play—*ai!*" Slowly the tears that a painful examination had not been able to stir now filled his eyes.

I patted the grubby little paw, and while he was being dressed, talked with the servant. "Carry him home and ask if his parents will let him stay in this hospital."

"If they do, Honorable Healer, may I stay with him?"

"No, but you may come to see him twice every day."

Torn by worry and devotion, the old fellow scratched his head over this problem of separation. "Always I have carried that Small One where he wished to go. It may be he will need me even in the Healing Hall."

"He will lie in a bed day and night; your work will be to come and tell him all that goes on in the street." After giving due consideration to this proposed change in duties, the coolie made no further protest.

When they were gone, I told my assistant, "Make arrangements with the child's people for him to enter at once, and find out what they can afford to pay."

"Suppose their silver is not enough, *Beh Ih-seng*, what then?"

"Then we shall find it somewhere else," I replied and turned to the next patient.

The following morning Lu Dih-dih entered the hospital. That he would have to endure much pain in order to gain his desire to move like other boys, I think he realized from that first day in dispensary. Our first problem was to build up his strength. Eggs, milk, and fruit were given him, and cod-liver oil in increasing doses. From the beginning he co-operated in every way, and the hospital attendants were soon his slaves. In a place of suffering high courage always commands tribute; when this quality is found in a child it becomes all the more remarkable.

"Good morning, *Beh Ih-seng*," was his usual greeting. "How are you? How is *Beh Si-mu?*"

"Well, thank you! And how is Lu Dih-dih today?"

"Two eggs I ate with my rice and two *dju-ger* (*Tu-hwa* for Mandarin oranges). Soon I will be a *pan tz* (fatty), not so? Look, Honorable Doctor, at my arm!"

Pinching the flesh that was gradually covering his bones, I would agree, "Truly, you are a *pan tz*."

This made him chuckle. "Also, I am very clean. Few people in Chungking are cleaner than I. Perhaps so much washing will make me thin again."

Together we laughed over this little joke. "Now, let's look at that leg."

His immediate response was to catch my free hand and hold it tightly until the nurse had once more replaced the covers. Often the bright black eyes were heavy with pain, but tears were not permitted to gather.

From the first he repeated the simple English phrases I used with the nurses when I was not sure of the Chinese words; then he would translate its meaning into the vernacular for my benefit. While this self-appointed teacher did nothing for my Mandarin, he did add enormously to my knowledge of Chungking earth-language.

Almost daily we surprised him with some trifle—a piece of foreign candy or a small slice of *dji dang gao* (high eggs) as the Chinese called our layer cake. One morning when the cod-liver oil had been increased to a quantity affecting appetite, Maud took him a stick of spearmint-flavored chewing gum to help clear away the oil odor and taste.

After the usual elaborate thanks, he removed the wrappings, then asked in a puzzled voice, "I eat this?"

"Yes, but remember not to swallow it!"

Late that afternoon he told me, "*Beh Si-mu* has a good heart. She brought me a sugar-thing. I liked it. Afterwards, I was hungry and ate all my midday food. Very strange! When I eat candy, I am not hungry."

Since the chewing gum seemed to solve the oil problem, I promised, "You may have a piece every morning and every afternoon."

This made him thoughtful. "I am most unworthy of such fine gifts," he protested with true Chinese courtesy, then pointing to blossoms in a bowl on his table, added, "Lao Er brought these miserable flowers from my home. Will you please carry them to *Beh Si-mu?*"

In three months he had gained so much I felt that an operation might be attempted. The flabby flesh had become firm and plump beneath a satiny skin, and the lines of suffering had almost completely disappeared from around eyes and mouth. I did not mention this plan in advance, being fully aware of all that the child had previously endured at the hands of native doctors.

Two of these local physicians, whose specialty was the treatment of bone tuberculosis, arthritis, and other

8

joint disturbances, conducted a place on a prominent street corner close by. Several times I had gone down there to watch them work on a victim.

First, with the place exposed, a square nail was driven into the flesh at what was supposed to be the focal point of infection. Rotating the nail between his hands, the doctor increased pressure until this crude instrument scraped the bone. The drilled opening was now enlarged in area, after which the nail was extracted and the blood permitted to flow. At the first sign of clotting, the physician spat saliva into the wound. In the Chinese interior, saliva was considered an excellent antiseptic, as it had been in some other ancient medical systems; indeed only for a generation or so have children in the West been taught not to suck sore fingers. A thick application of the greenish-black salve that the Chinese consider a panacea for all wounds and eruptions followed next and topping this, a piece of coarse tan fiber paper finished the dressing.

The Chinese are familiar with anesthesia, but I saw none used in these cases, and naturally the performance was torture for the patient. I managed to keep track of some of these after they went home and was amazed that so few infections resulted. The free bleeding was undoubtedly one reason. It was also quite possible that the salve used contained valuable healing properties.

The scars on Lu Dih-dih's hips told of several such operations; when I thought of them, the prospect of inflicting further pain in order to help the child was hard to face. On the scheduled day, the small patient was carried without warning into the operating room and there, holding to my hand as usual, he was put to sleep.

I opened the hip up widely, chiseled out all the decayed bone I could find and anchored what remained of the femur with wire to the pelvis. This made the repaired limb three to four inches shorter than the other, but was unavoidable. The boy stood the operation remarkably well, and within a few weeks seemed in fine shape.

Each morning now when I entered, he would ask, "Tomorrow do I walk?"

"Not tomorrow; perhaps in a few days."

His disappointment over these postponements was no greater than my own, for I had taken some liberties in that operation and I was anxious to see the leg in action. Also, I had felt for a long time that if I accomplished nothing else in China but to help this boy walk, the time would be well spent.

One morning when he had rested from his massage treatment, I walked into his room with two nurses and announced, "Lu Dih-dih, today you may try to stand."

His face was pale with excitement as the nurses lifted him from the bed, then stood supporting him on either side, while I pushed a wooden block under the short leg to give balance. For several seconds the small body swayed, then it crumpled. When I lifted him, he whispered as if overcome by shame, "*Beh Ih-seng*, I do not know how to use my legs."

"Lay down your heart! You will learn that quickly," I assured him, and after several attempts he stood erect.

Each day seemed to show improvement on the previous one; but just as I was ready to admit success, the site of operation began to drain. Repeated irrigations of Dakin's Solution achieved nothing, and a long, discouraging period of many months followed. I found it necessary again and again to reopen the wound, curette, and repack. Twice daily tuberculin paste was injected into the affected sinus tract. Why my young patient did not lose faith in that dark period, I never understood. The spark of determination to walk and to play seemed to burn at the center of his small being. In adults I had seen much brighter flames flicker and die before the fierce winds of pain. But in time healing occurred, and more than a year after he entered, Small Brother Lu was discharged from the hospital.

During the periods of convalescence between operations, I had sent him home several times for a few days' change. His parents, who had been unable to contribute anything toward their son's expenses, seemed grateful for what was being done, and each time he returned the boy brought little gifts to the attendants.

In that year, the old coolie became as much a part of our main corridors as one of the wicker chairs. One afternoon when he was ready to carry his charge into the sunshine of the yard, Lu Dih-dih asked, *"Beh Ih-seng,* many times has *Beh Si-mu* come to my room. May I go to your home to thank her?"

After this first trip—the house was only a few doors from the hospital—our residence became his most popular goal. Typical of his race, he never went empty-handed to a friend, and in preparation for these little visits, Lao Er would have brought flowers, or two pumelos (large citrus fruit resembling grapefruit), or several persimmons. Since the coolie was carrying him, the boy always insisted on using the servants' entrance, but before they left, he would ask to be carried to the front porch and placed in a chair. There he would sit for ten or fifteen minutes in quiet dignity, as if to announce to the world his intimacy with all under this roof.

When he was at last able to depend on his own feet—a high, cork-soled shoe had been made for the short leg—he soon became agile in manipulating the stiff hip. One day he surprised me beyond words by kneeling to kotow when he greeted me. This was a customary courtesy from Chinese children, but I had never expected him to master it. His joy was complete when the children in the neighboring day school permitted him to join them in tossing a tennis ball to and fro in their yard. That noon he waited for me outside our gate. "First I walk, *Beh Ih-seng,*" he told me, "now I play like other boys. As you promised, so it is."

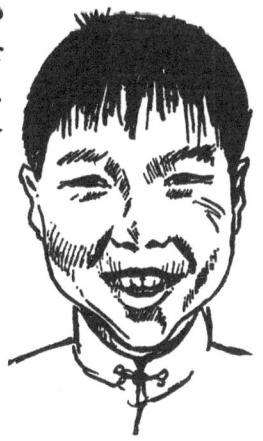

I had been afraid that association with those of his age might make him painfully aware of difference, but he showed none of this. Swinging leg and cork shoe had no power to dull his happiness, for this child who had always been dependent on others felt no need now to ask help of anyone.

A year or two later, in the days before I left Chung-king, Lu Dih-dih followed me about like a shadow. "When will you come back, *Beh Ih-seng?*" he would ask as he tendered another small gift for me to take to *Mei Gwu* (America—literally, The Beautiful Country).

"I do not know, Younger Brother. Perhaps when *Beh Si-mu* is well again."

At the moment of final good-by, he clung to my hand as he had done so often in the past. "You will not forget Lu Dih-dih?"

"No, Lu Dih-dih," I promised, "I'll not forget you. Whenever I think of China, I'll think of you." I might have added, "And at the thought of you, Small Brother, all of my China memories will be enriched."

Suddenly, with words at an end, tears welled in his eyes. Turning to the old coolie, that faithful refuge since infancy, he said, "My years are twelve, but I am still a baby. Lao Er, let us go home!"

CHAPTER VIII

The Military Throws a Few Rocks

Chinese abhor loneliness when ill, and this fact, more than any other, I believe, had contributed to the laxity previously existing in the hospital. Relatives and friends came and went at will in sick rooms, frequently remaining overnight and always bringing with them a supply of contraband foodstuffs. Ignorant of modern principles of hygiene and sanitation, most of these visitors treated the institution exactly as they did their own homes. I was congenitally opposed to operating a hospital along these lines, and I set about making changes at once. Their accomplishment required many months.

After the building had been disinfected and freshly painted from top to bottom, the most urgent of remaining problems was to establish a diet kitchen on each floor. Special stress was laid on the importance of keeping these rooms immaculate, and the first night after they went into use, I made unannounced inspection. My blood pressure shot up to a new high when I discovered that scraps from supper bowls had been thrown as usual on the floor, and I shouted for the coolie in charge.

"What did I tell you about these rooms?" I demanded.

"To keep them very clean, *Beh Ih-seng.*"

"Look at that food on the floor!"

"Yes, yes, Honorable Doctor, I see," he replied soothingly, "but it will stay there only until morning. Lay down your heart! Long before the nurses come to prepare breakfast, the floors will be scrubbed."

"This minute they will be scrubbed, not tomorrow," I declared. "Do you forget all the rats and cockroaches in this building?"

"Perhaps if I placed a little poison among these scraps," he suggested brightly.

I gave a long sigh. "No poison here! Clean up these floors immediately, and never let me find food on them again!"

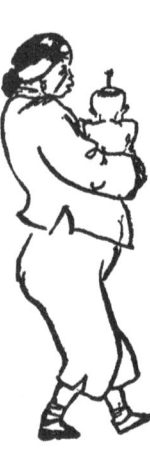

Like most coolies, he went off good-naturedly to get the bucket and mop, though he saw no good reason for doing so at the time.

Everything to do with food was a problem. We kept the nursery door locked not only as a safeguard against infections but also to prevent doting relatives from carrying out the babies for unscheduled feedings. Chinese think the practice of giving infants food only at stated intervals heartless in the extreme. A child nurses as often and over as long a period of time as it wishes; I have seen plenty of four- and five-year-olds still tugging at their mothers' breasts.

Difficulties were not limited to maternity cases. Families played fast and loose with diet restrictions, regardless of the patients' condition. To the Chinese, food is one of the most important things in life, and he who refuses to eat is reckoned ill indeed. In such a case it becomes the duty of relatives to tempt him with delicacies. Constantly we had to confiscate dishes brought in from the outside; it was even more troublesome to remove gifts of live fowls and fish from sick rooms. A few patients co-operated with the hospital willingly, but the majority resorted to all sorts of ruses in their smuggling enterprises.

The following letter from a young teacher in the high school illustrates this Chinese point of view.

My dear Doctor Basil:

This is to thank you for your skilful healing and kind treatment of my wife. Ever since she entered the hospital, she had been getting better day after day, until two or three days ago, she fell seriously again ill. My opinion should be that her recent falling sick is due to nothing but carelessness of food. For, having been sick for such a long time, she wanted very badly to take some delicate dish. How can we refuse to have her wish fulfilled, thinking she is so pitiable? Therefore we have supplied her from home some food, such as fish, chicken, and the like.

I write this to beg that you will be so kind as to cure her with what method you have used so effectually.

Yours sincerely,

Mei Yen-hsan

One day paying an unexpected visit to a patient on a non-protein, liquid diet, I noticed a strong odor of fish. While the nurse rearranged her pillows, my hands were busy exploring beneath the edge of the mattress, and almost at once, they came in contact with something which in my experience was quite foreign to hospital beds. Successively I pulled out a can opener and four small flat tins, now emptied of their original contents—sardines in mustard sauce. The woman stared at me with frightened eyes as I told her that a little more such nonsense might have killed her. Then carefully weighing the need for severe punishment, I forbade her all visitors for the rest of her stay in the hospital. Word of this dreadful example flew along the corridors, discouraging others with similar ideas.

The most trying phase of any doctor's experience in a field where fundamental theories of health are so diametrically opposed to his own, is that of never being able to relax supervision over details that in the West would be someone else's concern. One morning I happened to be standing by an open window above the kitchen yard when a vendor brought in two tins of water containing fish. To be salable in China, fish have to be swimming. These were apparently on their last strokes, for our cook, after one glance at them, resorted to most uncomplimentary remarks.

"Yes, a little sleepy," admitted the salesman, "but very cheap!"

"Naturally! Soon they will die."

"Lazy men live longest," philosophized the vendor. "It may be the same with fish."

"Do you think I was born yesterday? Already worms breed in them."

"What of it? At my price they are a gift." Abruptly he lifted his carrying-pole to position; adding, "Some other will buy them."

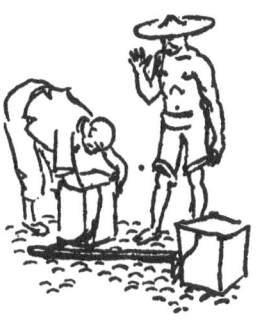

As he started off, the cook, succumbing to temptation, called him back and made the purchase.

Seeking the cook in the kitchen, I demanded, "Why did you buy bad fish?"

He wore an expression of startled innocence. "Not bad, *Beh Ih-seng*, only troubled with worms! I put them in the cistern and they seem reasonable. Soon they will be better, I think. If the Honorable Doctor wishes to taste them first when they are cooked, I . . ."

"How many times," I interrupted, "have I told you that bad food kills even strong people? Destroy those fish at once!"

"But I paid good silver for them, *Beh Ih-seng!*"

"That is your affair. Since you are so careless, perhaps the hospital should invite another cook to do your work."

I turned on my heel, fully aware that I would meet those fish again, in the accounts, disguised as meat or vegetables. No self-respecting *da-si-fu* (chief servant) was likely to pay out his money simply to satisfy a foreign doctor's foolish whim.

In the home Maud was having her own troubles along this line. Ordering clear soup one evening for dinner when guests were expected, she discovered on a hurried trip to the kitchen that the thick stock was being strained through a rag usually kept for scouring purposes. For the rest of her time in China she stuck to canned consommé.

Water, carried up from the river by coolies, went through a complicated process before it was ready for foreign home consumption. That which remained clear after alum had settled the Yangtze mud was filtered in sand, gravel, and green leaves. It was then boiled for another twenty minutes and filtered once more.

For hospital use the water had yet to be distilled and stored in sterile containers. By this time, robbed of all minerals and most gases, it had been reduced to H_2O, a liquid that could not quench thirst and that sometimes caused an unpleasant reaction in the patient, when injected intravenously. Unable to realize that they were endangering lives, the Chinese servants so frequently slipped up on these endless details of preparation that foreign supervision was essential.

I began to believe that Hercules had never faced a task comparable in difficulty to that of explaining germs to the average uneducated Chinese. Shrewd, ingenious, and tolerant, as I eventually found them,

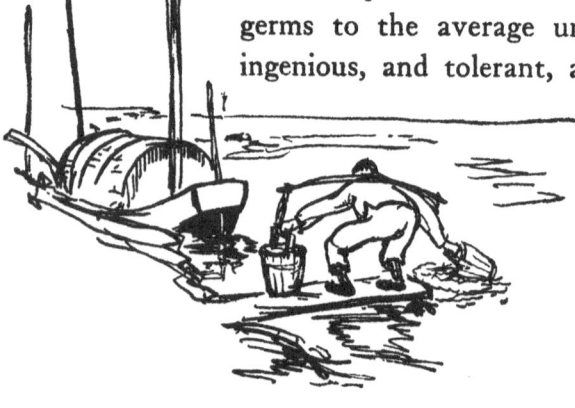

these people were willing to admit the possibility of much that was incredible. However, when one told them in all seriousness that millions of small harmful creatures existed in one drop of unboiled water, they remarked simply in their own tongue, "*Lan deh hsin!* (Too hard to believe!)" Moreover, they argued, when water was dirty, it had body; boiling took all the strength from it.

Once as I stressed the importance of sterile drinking water to a group of Chungking Middle School students, one stood up suddenly to ask, "Does *Beh Ih-seng* always drink skimmed milk?"

"Of course not," I replied promptly, falling into the pit he had prepared for me.

His shoulders shrugged expressively and with a glance that included all present, he questioned, "Then why skimmed water?" and sat down.

Aside from the demands of hospital routine, it seemed to me that I was compelled to spend more time worrying about the military faction than anything else.

As General Chang had promised, the members of his council came and in time brought families and friends. Far too many of these for my own peace of mind were in the army. As the Chinese expressed it, "A fool seeking trouble becomes the friend of generals." In our case the militarists did the seeking, but the result was the same. When an officer was admitted to the hospital, he brought with him the usual quota of

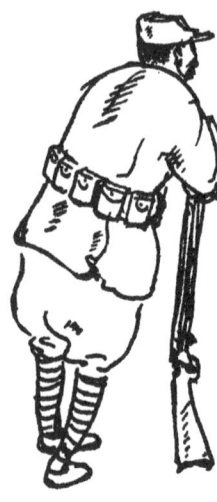

relatives and friends and a substantial bodyguard as well. Even after I had succeeded in making it clear— and this had to be done for each individual patient —that the sick alone could be accommodated, the uniformed men continued to loiter in corridors and get in everybody's way.

Through the ages the Chinese masses have asked only one thing of Life: to be permitted to work in peace. As long as the local official or village elder was even fairly good, the citizens concentrated on earning a livelihood and paid little attention to what was happening in higher government circles. This indifference has made them easy prey for politicians with a thirst for power and with troops at command. The Chungkingese living in a temptingly rich port were no exceptions to this rule. In order that the city might be saved for looting and for trade, most of the battles between opposing factions were fought a short distance away in the countryside.

Overlordship shifted from one general to another. While the *Tuchun* (Military Governor) in power was spending the city's confiscated revenues on gambling and concubines, his underlings attended to the business of government. The troops, meanwhile, were free to loot and, incidentally, to make life miserable for the inhabitants. Some of these soldiers were pathetic victims of circumstance, conscripted originally against their will, but the majority answered the old Chinese definition of warrior: *Muh iu shen mo yong chu* (utter worthlessness).

The major part of Szechuen, including Chungking, was at that time in the hands of a warlord named Den. A crafty politician and an able general, he had managed to stay in power for a number of years. His chief antagonists were a nephew of the same name and a General Wang. These two, working in co-operation, controlled the rest of the province and, unlike most warlords, were really concerned about the welfare of citizens in their territory.

Generalissimo Chiang Kai-shek, bent on adding Szechuen's allegiance to the Central Government in his program of national unification, now made overtures to the three of these leaders in the hope that they would patch up their differences. For a time there was no response. Then Wang, consulting with the nephew, made the first move. He arrived in Chungking.

To my great surprise he came straight to the hospital, explaining that his physical condition required some attention. I gave him a superficial examination but could find nothing the matter. Together we decided that a few days in the hospital under observation might be worth while, and he soon was occupying our best room.

Neither tests nor prolonged questioning—he seemed very hazy about symptoms—revealed more than had the office examination, and I was in a quandary. Here was one of the most important men in the province insisting on poor health while the doctor was equally certain that the patient was in excellent shape. To save "face" for both of us, I prescribed a mild tonic, at the same time admitting frankly that there was nothing more I could do for him. He accepted both medicine and statement with his usual dignity, then assured me that he was enjoying this rest in the hospital and would remain a few days longer.

From the first the Chungking papers had carried news of Wang's arrival and his stay at our hospital. Gossip was rife over the fact that he had come straight into Den's capital and, what was more, had brought a sizable retinue with him. Everyone knew that while the two generals had preserved a truce for a year or more, they had never yet sat down at a conference table together.

One morning Wang told me that he now felt quite rested and was leaving the hospital. After his departure I learned that Den had invited him to prolong his Chungking visit in order to discuss affairs of state. Suddenly the whole puzzle was solved. Wang, a real patriot anxious to achieve provincial unity, had made the first concession by coming to Chungking where Den was established. Much too shrewd to force the other's hand openly, he had chosen the excuse of hospitalization, not because of need, but to give Den opportunity for the next move in this Oriental chess game.

His presence in the city put the Chungking warlord "on the spot." That worthy, opposed to any movement that might limit his own power, had hoped to make Nanking believe that Wang was unwilling to co-operate; now to save his own face he must meet Wang halfway.

Surprisingly enough they managed to come to terms. Szechuen allied itself to the Central Government; Wang and the nephew achieved what they thought best for their people; and Den kept for his own the lion's share of Chungking customs duties and opium taxes.

General Wang remained in Chungking for a number of weeks, and I had occasion to see him once again— this time under tragic circumstances. He had a great many friends in the city, and the masses seemed to respect him beyond most militarists. There were two good reasons for this: First, he paid his soldiers a regular wage; second, he insisted on upholding the rights of citizens.

Between calls one midsummer afternoon, I stepped into a tea-house on a main thoroughfare and ordered a drink. Two petty officers sat at a table near by, and as I waited for my beverage to cool, they rose, belched loudly, and turned to leave, ignoring the youthful waiter who hurried forward with their bill. "Gentlemen," he called after them, "you have not yet paid!"

The soldiers gave no sign of having heard, and my own waiter, with what I considered a good deal of

9

courage, now joined the other in protest by reaching out and pulling at one offender's sleeve. Infuriated by this familiarity, the officer jerked his arm free and, swinging round, cuffed the boy brutally about the head. "This will teach you to respect your superiors!" he snarled, then started once more toward the entrance.

The commotion brought the proprietor and other servants to the scene and crowded the open front with interested spectators from the street. A Chinese gentleman garbed in satin, who had been sitting with a companion at an inconspicuous table, now pushed his way to the center of things and demanded sharply, "Pay what you owe!"

As he passed me, I recognized this successful-looking civilian as no other than my recent patient, General Wang. The note of authority in his voice halted the two soldiers, but without turning, the one who had beaten the waiter blustered, "This is our affair!"

His companion glancing back over a shoulder now paled to ghastliness. Frantically searching his money bag for coins, he whispered to the other, "Our General! Our General!"

From this moment terror held them both in its grip. When the account had been settled, General Wang continued with ominous calm, "As officers, you know the penalty for molesting civilians?"

"Yes, Your Excellency!"

"Your names?"

The answers came through dry lips.

"Now turn and face that wall!" he commanded, pointing to an empty space. When the two, obeying as if hypnotized, had done as directed, their commander drew a revolver from within his satin robe and put a bullet into each man's brain.

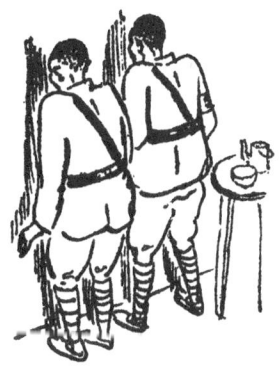

However horrifying such summary methods of justice may seem to the Westerner, the Chinese Military have no doubts about their efficacy. Once when I protested the execution of an innocent man, the official responsible for the death sentence admitted that the affair was sad but unavoidable. "For such a crime as this, an immediate example of punishment is necessary. Since we cannot find the guilty, some other must substitute. As a result, evildoers in this city will step more softly and many times one life may be saved."

My own first military tilt was with a colonel. He appeared one day at the hospital office and asked for a private examination. The routine charge for fee in advance was presented, but he refused to pay it. "I will give no doctor twenty-five dollars (ten in gold currency)," he announced flatly.

This charge insuring personal attention and complete privacy had been made especially for officialdom and the well-to-do who were unwilling to wait with the rank and file in dispensary and clinic. "In the dispensary, Sir," the clerk explained courteously, "you may be examined for two dollars."

"Then I will pay the foreign doctor two dollars to examine me in his office."

Aware of our Chinese personnel's timidity in dealing with soldiers, I suddenly appeared on the scene. "You wish to speak to me?" I asked.

"You are *Beh Ih-seng?* I came to be examined."

"I'll take care of you at once. The fee is twenty-five dollars," I reminded, pushing forward the same form he had refused. He paid without another word.

Just before entering my personal office, he halted, coughed, and spat on the floor. "If you wish to spit again, Colonel Chu," I suggested politely, "I feel sure you will not mind using the receptacle in the lavatory for that purpose." Then I called his attention to the immaculate appearance of the interior and expressed my appreciation of all that our patients and guests were now doing to help keep it so.

His only response was to stare at me in amazement, so I continued by way of explanation, "In America spitting on floors is considered dangerous to health, since many diseases are spread in that way." Then opening the door, I motioned for him to enter.

He did not move. "Always I spit where I wish," he said with a short laugh, "and I still live!" Deliberately he repeated the offense.

"If you do not wish to obey hospital rules, Colonel," I remarked quietly, "the office will gladly return your money."

"When I am in my home," he retorted, "I spit on the floor. When I am in the street, I spit on the street. When I am in this hospital, I spit in this hospital."

"In your home, Colonel, you may spit on the floor. On the street also you may spit, but in this hospital you must swallow your spit or leave."

"No!" he contradicted. "This hospital is on Chinese soil and I may do what I please. You are only a foreigner; while in this country you must do as *we* say."

I walked to the nearest hall window and pointed to the American emblem flying from its pole. "Do you see that flag?" I asked.

"Yes."

"It means that in this hospital you are on land that the Central Government permits my country to call its own, as long as we obey the laws."

"So?" He spat again, this time on the window sill.

A nurse passed at the moment, and I called out sharply, "Tell the clerk to send me the twenty-five dollars this officer just paid."

My visitor flushed. "You refuse to examine me?"

"In this institution all patients must obey rules," I answered. When the money arrived, I handed it to him and led the way to the open front entrance.

He followed slowly. On reaching the doorway, he challenged, "Suppose I do not wish to leave—what then?"

"You will leave just the same, Colonel Chu."

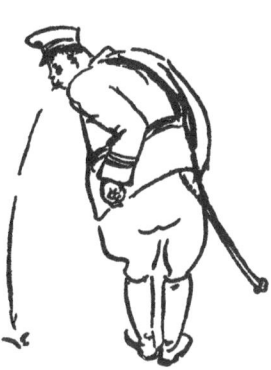

"Who will make me do so?"

"I will!" I snapped, now thoroughly angry, and gave him a push.

To my astonishment the thick-set, uniformed figure took a step forward, staggered, then rolled gracefully down the half-dozen steps to the walk. I started to his assistance, but realizing that this performance had been much too carefully managed to have harmful results, abruptly halted. For several moments he lay there moaning. Slowly pulling himself to his feet, his fury found expression. "For trying to kill an officer, Foreign Dog, you shall pay well! It is plain that you are one of the Communists who wish to destroy our people. I shall tell the *Tuchun* that and he will know what to do." Following this threat, he stalked down to the gate, bawled for his chair-bearers, and disappeared into the crowded street.

This was a great to-do, I thought ruefully as I re-entered the hospital. Although his fall had been swiftly staged, the fact remained that I had supplied an impetus. Resentment had landed me in an uncomfortable position, for it was not likely that the colonel would soon forget the affront or that he would forbear seeking vengeance.

The term, Communist, carried with it the greatest potential danger of the whole episode, for citizens of that persuasion in Chungking were in evil repute. Beheading attended discovery of anyone supposed to

have such political affiliations, and many innocent had
perished with the guilty.

Even to be associated with one meant death. A
month or so earlier, on my way to Dsen Gia Ngai, I
had come upon a gathering outside the City Wall, and
always curious about such throngs, had joined it.
Three soldiers were standing in a cleared space,
spinning an abject individual round and round like
a top.

Faster and faster the poor wretch whirled. Puzzled,
I asked a bystander, "What queer affair is this?"

"They would kill that Communist."

"He's no Communist," muttered a farmer in from
the fields. "He showed pity to one in hiding and for
that he dies. A great business indeed!"

Several others near by eyed the countryman with
suspicion and one suggested, "Perhaps you are one of
them."

"Not so!" came hotly. "But is it Chinese custom
to kill men for having good hearts?"

In the new wave of excitement, this humble advo-
cate of freedom was forgotten. One of the soldiers had
whipped out a sword and with a single stroke cut off
his prisoner's head. It was doubtful whether the poor
fellow even knew of this last indignity, for his over-
taxed heart must already have failed him. The head
was next paraded through the streets on a pole, then
erected in the only parklike square the city boasted.

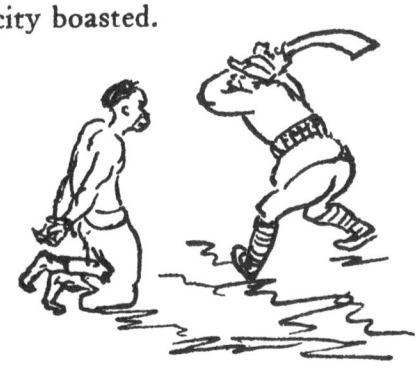

On my following trip to the country, a week later, the swollen, headless corpse still lay where it had first fallen. Putrefaction and dogs had both made their inroads, but no man had dared to touch it, fearing similar punishment. I heard later that some sorrowing connection of the dead had placed two dollars on what remained of the body, and overnight it was removed for burial, probably by some outcast so desperate for the silver that life seemed a small risk in exchange.

Usually Communists were executed in groups, first suffering the shame of being marched through the streets and then shot one by one. This course forced all but the first to taste death many times through their comrades. After such mass executions, coolies would go down to the scene and dip coins in the pools of blood—these to be used as amulets against Communistic influences.

Where foreigners were concerned, persecution had come chiefly from Communists themselves and not from anti-Communists. For a period of several years the Revolutionists had cut a deep swathe of suffering wherever they passed, spilling the blood of "foreign imperialists" impartially with that of their own race.

Later, after the Japanese war broke out, the scattered remnants of the once powerful and merciless Red Army, together with all other political parties in China, swore allegiance to the Central Government. Then it swiftly became the fashion to glorify the famous "Communist" trek to the Northwest and to criticize Generalissimo Chiang Kai-shek for ever having wasted the nation's time and resources fighting the revolutionists. To argue along this line is to forget the bitter years of Communist uprisings, with the futile and unnecessary destruction of private life and property that lay in the wake of revolutionary progress.

Today, it is true, those same so-called "Reds" are contributing magnificently toward national salvation; also their once pure and unadulterated Russian theories have become so pale a pink that unprejudiced observers find them closely resembling democratic ideals. But the fact remains that there was a day, and not long since, when the red flag in China was a symbol of terror, and the young Central Government, endeavoring to develop a constructive program, was forced either to conquer these latest rebels against law and order or to perish at their hands.

Chungking had experienced its own Communist scares. During my residence, the city was without a United States Consul, so a government gunboat was usually anchored offshore to act as a court of last resort for Americans in difficulty. Registrations, passports, and the like were all transacted by mail with the American Consulate in Hankow, a thousand miles down river; but in everything else affecting "Uncle Sam's" citizens, "Navy" represented Washington.

Early one morning a chit-coolie (note bearer) from the gunboat brought the following letter:

United States Asiatic Fleet
Yangtze Patrol
U. S. S. ———

Chungking, China
19 April, 19—

To: All United States Citizens Present.

The Commanding Officer has received information which indicates that Communists are planning disturbances throughout China on 20 April (Monday). The apparent object is to attack foreigners and foreign property for the purpose of causing difficulties for the Central Government.

The local authorities are well aware of the plan and state that they have taken all precautions and that they do not expect any serious trouble. However, they advise all foreigners, and I advise you, to be extremely careful to avoid difficulties with Chinese, especially from April 19 to April 22, inclusive. The Chinese authorities further advise that foreigners living far from shore on the South Bank move closer in before the night of April 20.

Due to the fact that Americans and American subjects are so widely separated in this vicinity, it will be impossible for this vessel to furnish armed forces for protection ashore.

However, anyone who desires to come aboard the ——— will be gladly taken care of.

It is my personal opinion that no great disturbance can take place in this vicinity and that anything that may occur will be limited in extent.

Lieutenant Commander, U. S. N.
Commanding U. S. S. ———
Senior U. S. Naval Officer Present

There was some disturbance, but no tragic results in connection with this particular incident. However, it added still another straw to the local government's flame of indignation against the movement, and as is true of all such affairs, many innocent suffered with the guilty when punishment was officially meted out.

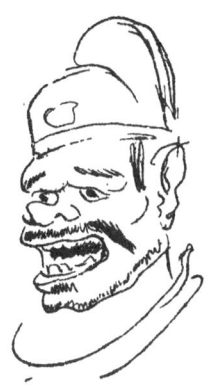

My head, belonging as it did to an American, was in no great danger as far as I could see; but for my name to be connected with the organization might prove ruinous to the hospital's future in the community.

As I had expected, Colonel Chu kept his word. During the next few days several small riots were staged in our compound to the accompanying yells, "Foreign Devil!" and "Communist!" but aside from a broken window or so, no real damage was done. Our official contacts were standing us in good stead, for there were repeated rumors that Colonel Chu was doing everything possible to have me deported.

My greatest annoyance arose from an article in a Shanghai paper. This stated that a foreign physician of Communist sympathies in Chungking had knocked an army officer down the steps of the institution, injuring the man seriously. In retaliation the hospital had been the scene of dreadful rioting, which had wrecked the building and harmed a number of patients. I was worried, more than I admitted even to Maud by this garbled publicity, but in a few weeks the excitement died down. Strangely enough, the unpleasant advertising increased patronage. Visitors now appeared for the sole purpose of seeing the place where not only ordinary people were expected not to spit but where even the military could be thrown out for doing so.

Three months passed before I saw the Colonel again. I was on my way to a patient's home, accompanied by her close friend, one of our American women teachers. Good custom dictated that men and women neither walk nor talk together on Chinese streets, and, for the sake of appearance, the average foreigner usually tries to observe native propriety in such matters. My companion and I, however, were so engrossed in discussing the prospective case that our progress was not strictly according to convention. My first intimation of this faux pas came when a man leaned toward my associate, suddenly hissed, "*Yang po tz!*" (foreign harlot), and spat.

He proved to be Colonel Chu indulging in his favorite habit. A few steps behind was his companion, a Chinese woman whose flamboyant makeup and lavish display of jewels labeled her a courtesan. Instantly I retorted with a similar epithet from my Chinese vocabularly. My antagonist glared, then moved on—apparently out of spittle for the moment.

Horrified by my having stooped to the Colonel's methods, the American woman rebuked me with the question, "Do you think that was wise, Doctor? You'll only make enemies, I fear."

"Wait and see!" I told her. "He knows we wouldn't permit another foreigner to insult one of our women that way—why should he be free to do so? No one respects a doormat, and these Chinese less than most people."

More months passed and one day a young officer presented himself for examination. "Colonel Chu sent me," he explained.

I stared. "*Who* sent you?"

"Colonel Chu," he repeated. "I am on his staff. He said you would tell me the truth about myself."

I made no further comment, except to inform him that he was the victim of gonorrhea in an advanced stage. From time to time other patients came in with the same introductory speech, and I wondered if the Colonel had experienced old-fashioned religious conversion.

When he appeared in person one day with an advance receipt for the twenty-five dollar fee, I decided Life held no more surprises.

"I wish to be examined, Doctor," he announced. After I had politely agreed, he added with a roguish expression, "Today, *Beh Ih-seng*, I hope that you will be able to accomplish more." Aware of the implications of this remark, we both burst into laughter.

As he stripped, I asked curiously, "Why did you send me those patients? Certainly it was not for friendship's sake."

"Truly not!" he explained. "I sent them for the same reason that I myself am here. A Chinese doctor always fears three things—the *Feng-shui* (elemental spirits), the patient's family, and the patient. Naturally, to keep from offending everybody he seldom tells the truth. What you fear, Foreign Doctor, I do not know, but I am sure it is none of these. Therefore, I am here!"

Later he told me frankly that he had always resented foreigners and all their ways. He had come to the hospital the first time only because of worry about his condition and of my recommendation from an acquaintance. My stubborn attitude about spitting had seemed rude and childish to him. In response, he had been very rude himself, and it was not until the unpleasant meeting on the street, when I had dared to return his insult, that he had worked out this personal theory about my professional use.

I found such candor highly interesting, and for the rest of his stay in Chungking we continued on the most amicable of terms.

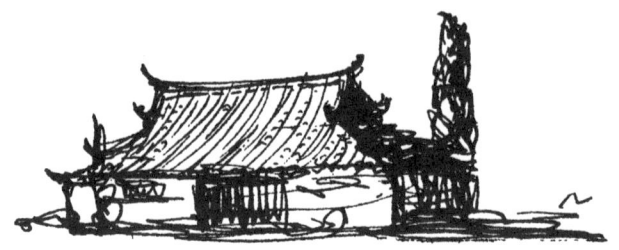

CHAPTER IX

A Study in Contrasts

Since I was the only foreign physician on the staff, my recreation was limited to odd times and places. At the hospital I was on twenty-four hour call, and the civic authorities had granted me a pass permitting me to be on the streets at any time of night, a privilege not accorded the average citizen.

Births, as every doctor knows to his sorrow, have a way of occurring between midnight and dawn. After one of these cases I was usually too wide awake to retire. Instead, slipping through the gateway I would find, in sharp contrast to the battle and clamor of daylight, a Chungking whose mysterious, black silence challenged me to exploration.

My shoes, rubber-soled, made muffled footfalls on the worn flagstones, and I could approach so quietly through the darkness that the guards drowsily patrolling thoroughfares were at times as startled by my sudden appearance as if I had been an apparition from some Taoist Hell. Although many of them had met me before, they would retaliate for these little surprises by gruffly demanding my pass and then stand there turning

131

it over and reading it upside down and backwards while we pursued the following sort of conversation.

"You are the doctor from the American Hospital, not so?"

"As it is written."

"Where do you go? And on what business?"

"No business—to walk on the street."

The rays from their small lantern cast eerie reflections on our faces, and I could watch, with inward amusement, their rapid exchange of glances, puzzled, questioning, stern.

"At the Hour of the Ox, it is not Chinese custom to be on the street."

"Truly? It is my custom."

The finality of this statement always seemed to impress them. The only way to deal with one so odd, they must have decided, was to give him his way. "*Ko ee!*" someone would suddenly agree, and with the pass safe again in my pocket, I moved on. It might have been enlightening, I used to think, to hear what was said after my departure.

"*Hsi chi deh hen!*" one might have exclaimed. "That healer's home in Dai Gia Hang has soft foreign beds, yet this late he is on the street. Also, he has silver to pay coolies and a fine chair of his own, but he walks. Why is this?"

"Who can say? All day he works in the *ih yuen*—does he never sleep?"

"Too hard to believe! We who watch at night must sleep in the day, *hsi puh hsi?*"

"Naturally. Not until the Hour of the Monkey do I rise and go to Wen's tea-house for a game. Pity the man who wakes me earlier!"

"All foreigners are queer, but this American more than most—*ai-ya!*"

Equipped on these strolls with flashlight and walking stick, I accounted for a good many killings in Chungking's rat colony. These rodents, as large as well-developed kittens, crossed the path at almost every step. Hunting them contained a dash of real sport, for night dew and mist made the flagstone streets even more slippery than in daytime, and then it was precarious enough. To my rubber soles the ooze gradually fastened like wet glue, and each sudden move on my part became a test of skill in retaining balance. On the other hand, the rats suffered the handicap of being temporarily blinded by the flashlight rays; and while they hesitated, thwacks from my cane dispatched them to some "happy hunting-ground" for rodents.

On either side, the narrow, winding streets were lined by tightly boarded shop-fronts or, in the residential sections, by high plastered walls in which an occasional dark wooden door served as entrance. At periodic intervals within the grounds watchmen swung harsh wooden rattles to denote that all was well. Barred against the world the Chungkingese, rich and

10

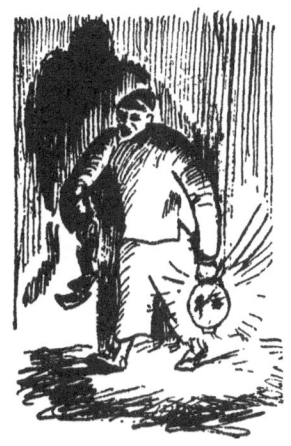

poor alike, slept and dreamed and in the morning woke to their scheduled appointments with tears or laughter.

The barking of a distant dog would find its echo close by in a hollow cough from some tubercular victim's tightly closed room. Occasionally where the wooden panels of a building had warped, a crack of light penciled a yellow line on the opposite street wall. Usually such illumination at this hour told of tense figures absorbed in a game, and if I paused to listen, the click-clack of dominoes could easily be heard. For the most part, though, Chungking's night ways were silent.

At such moments I wondered how many of these West China people slept peacefully. Was it possible that in the house to my right or in the one across the alley, someone tormented by pain or worry lay awake waiting for the long hours to pass? Already I had met personally some of the more unhappy members of this community.

Through one dark lacquered gate, there had come an emergency call to pump poison from the stomach of an eighteen-year-old daughter of the house. She was the sacrificial victim in a pathetic story, as old as Life itself. In love with a youth her own age and facing imminent marriage with an older suitor chosen by her parents, she had preferred to die. Two weeks after her recovery from this abortive attempt at suicide, the wedding had occurred as planned, and at odd moments the girl's hopeless expression continued to haunt me.

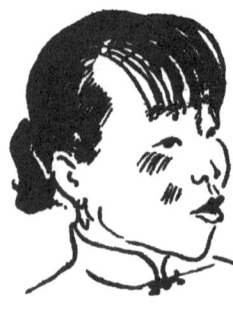

In a poorer quarter a woman, who had failed repeatedly in her consuming desire to carry a child through to maturity, was willing her own death in another way. Her husband had brought her to dispensary, saying, "She can eat nothing. I thought the foreigners might have a medicine for this ill."

Frequently syphilis is to blame for a series of miscarriages, and a Wassermann test is in order. This woman, however, proved to be suffering from anemia and malnutrition only, so I prescribed a good tonic and ordered an increased diet.

"Why should I waste silver on more food? Already I have lost four little ones. You did not understand, Doctor? Of four, *none* lived," reiterated the patient.

"Naturally—you are very weak. Build strength and you may have better fortune."

Her lips twisted bitterly. "The gods close their ears to my prayers—even Kuan Yin is deaf. I was strong enough with the first two, but they died also. It was the same with my mother; I was her only child who lived. *Mi teh fa!*"

I took the husband aside. "Your wife wishes to die. Why not adopt a son?"

"I thought of that plan but, no, she says I must have children of my blood. Had I enough silver, I would take a second woman under the roof—as it is, *liao puh deh!* (Impossible!) She is a good wife," he added, his brow furrowed with worry, "and I would rather have her than some other."

I saw this patient only once more and that by accident. She was evidently succeeding in her intention, for she looked almost ready for that grave her own hands had dug. Ever more often as time passed was I to be baffled by the differences in Oriental and Occidental ways of thinking. Raw emotions were much the same the world over—in the thought processes stimulating these lay the mystery.

Alone, and close to the city's beating heart in this nocturnal prowling, I could feel Chungking's peculiar quality wrap itself about me like a cloak. During most of her many centuries of history no pink-skinned foreigners had trod these ancient thoroughfares; even today their presence was tolerated, not desired. And yet I had the feeling that the city, accustomed to agelong conquest, set herself determinedly to win even the alien and "the barbarian" within her gates. What, I asked myself frequently, is the secret of her fascination? Bemused by these thoughts, I would make my way home and there drop instantly into dreamless sleep.

While Chungking and her people were gradually absorbing my interest, the foreigners in her midst demanded their own share of attention. All types of individuals and representatives of many races made up the groups of missionaries and business people. At first

I found it hard to understand why so many barriers separated the two sets of foreigners. Later, becoming more familiar with their conflicting ideologies and purposes, I saw that some differences were bound to arise; but my conviction that many of these were artificial and, therefore, unnecessary, still remains. Altruism had undoubtedly prompted the presence of most missionaries on the field. It was equally true that the business people could claim no motive more virtuous than commercial instinct to account for their own appearance there. But these simple premises seemed insufficient to explain all the intolerance some members of each group held for those of the other.

In the intimacies peculiar to medical practice, I soon discovered that each camp had its share of good and bad. For the foreigner, prolonged residence in the Orient is an acid test of character—to remain normal in an abnormal environment is difficult indeed, and that all do not succeed is hardly a matter for wonder.

Of the two foreigners for whom I had the deepest respect in Chungking, Doctor Merton, a quiet, elderly English missionary whom everybody admired, was one; the other, Doctor Strobel, was considered by both missions and community "beyond the pale."

Once in a while one encountered a typical "Soldier of Fortune," like Parnell, who lived in our home for a number of months. Foreign houses are scarce in the interior of China, and paying guests are apt to apply wherever there is room to receive them. By that method Parnell arrived under our roof. Just over thirty, he had jumped from one adventurous experience to another. From the latest of these, a dangerous enterprise in North China, he had landed into what must have seemed to him a very prosaic business—selling a foreign production in Chungking.

Already in his brief career, he had made, lost, and laughed off three or four fortunes. His charm was like quicksilver, and chit-coolies bearing social invitations were always on his heels. He could "get away with murder" as the saying goes, not only among his own kind, but also with the Chinese, who are usually too shrewd to be easily fooled. What made this even more surprising was the fact that Parnell knew almost nothing of the language, an important key for the purpose of unlocking their friendship. By using a half-dozen simple phrases, he managed, to everyone's amazement, to transact business successfully throughout the whole of Szechuen Province.

At that time Chungking, with its numerous streets of steps, seemed the least likely place on earth to use an automobile. Yet Parnell contrived to negotiate not only the occasional narrow level, but he actually forced a machine to go up and down Djiu Iu Gai (Nine-Step Alley) outside our compound.

In these amazing experiments he was always immediately surrounded by curious, frightened spectators, and once in trying to turn the car, he crushed a child against a wall. For almost any other foreigner, this accident would have meant disaster, but not for him. Leaving the vehicle where it was, he caught the boy up in his arms and brought the unconscious figure, with its shattered leg dangling against his body, straight to the hospital. I saw at once that amputation was unavoidable; and only after many weeks did the child recover sufficiently to go home. Meanwhile, Parnell had been hard at work appeasing the parents, and they did not even sue him for damages, although their son was doomed to be a cripple throughout life.

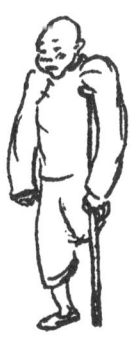

Tales of this sort made the man an almost fabulous figure in the community. Whenever anything unusual occurred, it became the custom to ask, "Was Parnell there?" He had no flagrant vices. Women found him particularly attractive, but he handled all such matters with adroitness. One drink was usually his limit, and under that slight stimulation he talked at his best. In conversation he was quite as likely to discuss the genius of Edgar Allen Poe as some gilt-edged proposition that would make one rich for life. If the first, one knew a great deal more about ravens when he finished than when he began.

Every once in a while, though, the Chinese, with their unbeatable business acumen, would trip him up in a deal. For a day or so Parnell would go about grimly, then with a swift resumption of self-confidence, he would say, "George, I've got a new idea! I'll get every cent of that money back yet."

But I doubt if he did, although occasionally he made a surprising scoop. Dave was clever beyond most of us, but the Chinese were past masters in the same field, and few people have every lived who could lick them more than once in financial deals.

As is so often true of the world's charmers, being his intimate had one disadvantage—he was likely to impose on good nature. T——, our mutual friend and an admirable young business man, let himself become "the goat" for Parnell's ideas, sometimes at the sacrifice of personal comfort and convenience. Yet in an emergency, Dave could be counted on with the best. In one experience of my first year, he adapted himself readily to a situation so gruesome that most men would have refused bluntly to have anything to do with it.

Some ancient Greek is credited with the statement that "humor is the best test of gravity, and gravity of humor." Certainly Life has a way of working comic relief into the most horrible tragedies. Never before nor since this particular incident, have I had any experience that surpassed it for size or dreadfulness and yet, in my memory, the entire affair is linked with absurdities.

Just below the city wall at the rear of the hospital was an arsenal that manufactured high explosives.

The Chinese were adept at making the most complex firecrackers, but their attempts to copy modern Western projectiles presented real problems. In the Chungking arsenal at that time there was no regulated system of grading what went into the shells, and one bomb might be several times as powerful as another of the same size. To overcome this, these munitions workers used a testing method that must have been unique even for the Orient. Taking a sample of a composition, they would pack it into a small shell case and explode this by fuse right on the earthen floor of the factory, while the workmen stood about only a few yards away. As might be expected where the calculations in dealing with explosives were guesswork, fatalities were bound to occur. This time the whole arsenal blew up.

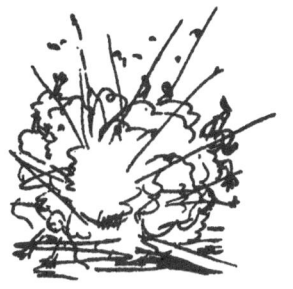

Arriving home at dusk, I had sat down for a few minutes of reading before dinner. Szechuen, as usual, was experiencing provincial strife, and reverberation of guns was common. Naturally, when the windows rattled about me, I paid no attention, until a servant rushed in to announce excitedly, "*Beh Ih-seng*, soldiers fight and the hospital is filled with wounded."

Such news, bringing the inevitable complications of military patients, gave me a headache. Laying down my journal, I rose lazily, ordered the servant to tell Mrs. Basil that I would be back shortly, and went out. In the gateway Parnell was just entering. "Hello," he sang out, "where are you going at dinner time?"

"To look at some wounded soldiers."

"I'll walk over with you."

Together we turned into the hospital grounds and there found bedlam. Everywhere injured men were crying and groaning. A few of these were in sedan-chairs, but the majority lay on the ground. Several were already dead, and I could not help but think them fortunate when I saw the awful condition of the living. The entrance corridor of the building was even more crowded with sufferers than the yard.

"What under heaven has happened?" I demanded of the first nurse I met. "Did they have the battle here in our compound?"

"No battle, *Beh Ih-seng*," she replied, "the arsenal just exploded." The girl's face was twitching, and afraid that she might add to difficulties by fainting, I issued a sharp order. "Place a servant temporarily in charge of each floor and get every other attendant in the building down here at once!"

The need for action restored her morale and she went off to her job. Caught shorthanded, I stood there for a second trying to figure the best way to handle this emergency. One of the Chinese internes was representing us at a medical conference in Peiping; the other was enjoying his night off in the Hills. There was no time to seek other doctors in the city; these probably had their own share of wounded. With treatment stations arranged for first-aid all along the hall, I

pointed out some of the most urgent cases and ordered
them brought to me in the emergency room on the
main floor.

This, always kept in readiness, contained two operating tables. As I scrubbed and slipped into a gown,
I turned to Parnell, who, undaunted by carnage, was
still with me. "Dave," I began slowly, "dozens of
arms and legs will have to be amputated. Alone I can
take care of a limited number; if you will watch me
on the first ones, you will be equal to helping with
some of the others."

He stared at me as if I had gone crazy, but nothing
"feazed" him for long. Biting down hard on the half-
smoked cigar between his teeth, he pulled off his coat
and turned to the basin. After a little time he started
on his own, sawing awkwardly—he was left-handed—
on the bodies I turned over to him with a few simple
directions. Together we soon filled several bamboo
baskets with dismembered limbs, and the blood on the
floor made footing difficult.

Occasionally I remembered to steal a glance at my
assistant to see how his nerves were holding up under
this surprising test. A frown knitted his brows and
perspiration rolled down his face, but he kept steadily
at the job, endlessly chewing his cold cigar, which was
certainly a strange property for a surgeon. Between
patients, he would call out through the other corner
of his mouth, "How am I doing, Doc?"

While I worked, I was painfully aware that there was little hope of saving many of these poor, tortured victims of the accident. For that matter recovery with a mutilated limb made life, itself, seem a questionable gift. In a land like China, where the problem to survive at all calls for unceasing struggle, the cripple is shown no quarter.

It was when my spirits were at lowest ebb that Grim Humor took a still more active hand. Into the middle of this scene of disaster casually sauntered my wife. By the time she arrived, all the bodies had been removed from the yard. The main corridor did seem to have an unusual amount of activity, Maud later admitted, but she had managed to walk right through the building into the emergency room before she became fully aware of what was going on. Once inside, however, she stopped abruptly halfway between door and operating tables. With a wild expression, her eyes took in the pool of blood on the floor, the spattered wall, my stained whites, and the incredible spectacle of Parnell sawing at a man's thigh. Then lifting a small yellow paper in one shaky hand, she seized a momentary lull to treble hysterically, "You were both so late for dinner that I thought I'd better bring over this wire for Dave."

At that moment there was no one on earth I wished less to see than Maud. The sight of even a few drops of blood had always bothered her; she was having trouble becoming acclimated, and our first child was due in three months. Yet there she stood extending her silly little slip of paper.

"Get out of here!" I yelled. "Get out!"

Without a word, much like a mechanical toy that had just been re-wound, she turned around and made her way homeward.

Several hours later Parnell and I joined her. Dinner was still waiting, and as the food disappeared, my wife's distaste for our appetites became increasingly obvious. "I've long since ceased being surprised by anything doctors do," she remarked, "but how you can eat a morsel tonight, Dave, is beyond me. If you could have seen yourself—oh!" She squeezed her eyelids as if to shut out the memory.

Parnell, to my surprise, seemed about to express himself seriously, then prompted by his usual perversity, gave me a sly grin. "I worked harder for this dinner," he protested plaintively, "than for any in years," and reaching out, he took a second piece of cake.

My wife eyed him coldly. "You're all alike," she said in a tone that washed her hands of masculinity in general. "And to think," she added as we rose from the table, "that I went into that awful, awful place just to see that you got your old cable promptly. Next time . . . !" Leaving this dire threat unfinished, she dismissed us with a shrug and left the room.

CHAPTER X

Enter the Feng-shui

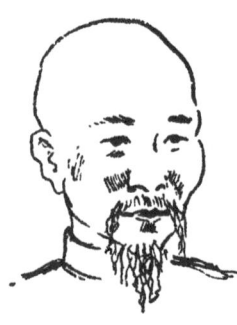

The Chinese language is a fascinating one. It is also tantalizing for those foreigners whose hours of study are limited. I had an excellent personal teacher, an old scholar who had taught many foreigners through the years; my problem was to find time for him. Some of the hospital staff had a fair knowledge of English; others knew only the simplest rudiments, and it became imperative that I learn to bridge the gap between these and myself.

To be a good guesser is a part of the standard equipment for a doctor anywhere; for the foreign medical man in China it is an essential. On arrival he is confronted by a language in which verbal and written symbols seem to have little in common and where one sound may stand for a variety of meanings, depending entirely upon the inflection used. Naturally this system presents an extraordinarily fertile field for development of errors. Cold chills used to play about my spinal column at the thought that life or death might depend on ability to comprehend verbal reports and to give clear directions. Not until my return to practice

in the States, where no language barriers existed between patient and physician, did I realize fully the
strain under which work in Chungking had been done.

In his later seventies when we knew him, Sung Lao Si,
our teacher, was a striking figure. Tall, spare, dignified, with a face that was beautiful in its serenity,
he impressed one immediately as a man of character.
He typified, I think, the fine qualities that are to be
found in so many of China's old-fashioned scholars.

That first summer in the Hills he came to us regularly
for several hours each day, and there, in a quiet study,
he strove to teach my wife and me the rudiments of
Mandarin, *a la* Szechuen. For the new arrival who can
spend his whole first year in a regular language school,
the problem of acquiring native speech is simpler than
for those who start right in on a regular job and
get their studying done on the side with a personal
teacher.

Sung Lao Si spoke no English, and in the end this
was best for us as students. We labored so hard to
understand what he was trying to say that our minds
gradually developed an extra-sensory alertness for
strange sounds. Tones or inflections are exceedingly
important in Szechuenese, and for the first six or eight
weeks of study the student simply does not hear them.
Indeed, he finds it difficult enough to catch the unfamiliar consonant tie-ups without bothering about
inflections.

Our lessons would start with an exchange of morning greetings, usually, "Sung Lao Si, *tsao!*" (Sung Scholar, Good-morning!)

"*Beh Ih-seng, tsao!*"

"*Beh Si-mu, tsao!*"

Then having done the right thing by the courtesies, the teacher would lose no time attacking our pronunciation of the word *tsao*. "*Dzow!*" he would say.

"Zow!" Maud and I would both repeat.

"*Puh!* (No!) *Dzow!*"

This often would go on a half-dozen times; then it would dawn on one of us that the word had a *d* sound, and the game was ours.

"This is what thing?" would be the next question in Chinese, as he held up a pencil or pointed to some other object in the room.

Maud and I would struggle painfully to get both sounds and tones correct in the simple answer, and then we would be defeated by using the wrong numerary adjunct, for each noun in Chinese has a special descriptive article of its own. For example, to say, "one box, one pen, one chair, one man," requires four different articles before the four nouns. Respectively these are: *ih-ko, ih-fen, ih-bah, ih-go.*

If the strain seemed to make temporary nervous wrecks of us, it must have been much worse on Sung Lao Si. He had dealt for a lifetime with the oddities and stupidities of adult foreign students, but now age was upon him, and the old man could stand only so much. A sincere Christian, who had first been disciplined in the Confucian school, he resorted to neither raised voice nor scolding words when the going became too rough. Instead, he would stop short, place one hand over his eyes, and say quietly, *"Ngo men iao tsu da gao!"* Following· this announcement he would talk out loud in Chinese, then abruptly resume the lesson.

For perhaps two months this happened at least once daily, but Maud and I had no clue to what it meant. Then one Sunday morning as Sung Lao Si conducted services in the hospital, I heard him use the familiar phrase. The action that followed gave me a clear translation. It was, "Now let us pray!"

As time passed, the old gentleman found it necessary to pray less often in the middle of lessons. The day eventually came when to stick an *h* between *t* and *sa*, in the aspirated *t'sa*, (Szechuenese for "tea"), was almost second nature. Words were now labeled in the mind with the numbers 1, 2, 3, and 4 to indicate tones. Whether one pitched a sound in high or low ranges, or gave it a graceful center curve depended entirely on the figure attached to it in the memory. Mixing these, or similarities in vowel sounds, led to numerous difficulties. By the merest vocal shift, one could change the meaning of the sound, *tso* (sit), for instance, to *tseo* (walk).

11

When, as soon happened, I took on full-time work at the hospital, my studying had to be done on the run. Sung Lao Si now followed me about the building, teaching whenever a spare moment could be found. Sometimes he would accompany me on local professional calls, and as we made our way together through the crowded streets, we would discuss a variety of subjects. As my vocabulary increased, I found him a delightful companion. There was little he did not know about his fellow Chungkingese, and he gave me a great many interesting sidelights on their way of life.

The citizens on their part paid the utmost respect to this austere old figure, garbed in long cotton gown and short black sateen jacket, with a round skull cap to match. He had accepted the foreigners' religion in his youth, when to do so meant not only ostracism from his own kind but the risk of life itself. For the sake of that conviction, he had endured much, and whenever I looked at him, I realized that his expression of serenity had grown from suffering and strife rather than peace. The Chinese respect virtue above all things, and while there were few Chungkingese who saw eye to eye with Sung Scholar on the foreign doctrine, they paid him unstinting tribute for his great qualities.

My time with Sung Lao Si was so limited and the necessity to learn quickly so pressing, I grasped at every word I heard. Many of these were picked up on the street from shopkeepers, passers-by, chair-coolies, and boatmen. As each new phrase reached my ears, I would repeat the sounds over and over to get rhythm, then store them in memory for future use. Sometimes I remembered to ask my teacher the meaning of these expressions; often I would just base interpretation on the way they had been used. As might be imagined, this second method had risks.

One afternoon I crossed on a Yangtze ferry with a boatman I had never before seen. He collected the customary fare of a few coppers from the other passengers but on reaching me, the only foreigner aboard, he demanded a dollar.

"A dollar!" I repeated. "Do you think I was born yesterday?"

"One dollar!" he reiterated truculently.

"The regular fare for one, that much I will give you, no more," I told him and held out the coins.

Gruffly pushing my hand aside, a most unusual rudeness for a Chinese, and thrusting his face close to mine, he began to express himself at length about "foreign dogs" and all their ways. Much of this speech was beyond me, but there was no mistaking the insulting tone and manner.

When he finally paused for breath, I asked, "Have you had your 'faceful'?" Several passengers tittered over this use of idiom, and the ferryman became angrier. Before he could resume the quarrel, though,

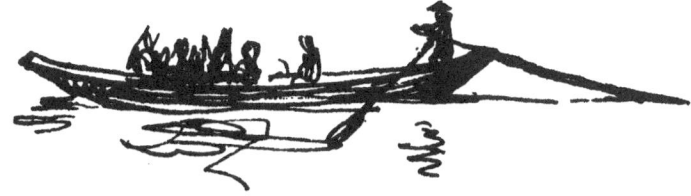

I proceeded with further personal remarks of my own. Amazingly enough, I soon found phrase after phrase rolling from my tongue. Where they came from and what they meant, were beyond me at the moment, but I had no doubts about their fitting the occasion. The effect on the audience proved nothing less than astonishing. Many stared open-mouthed, and my adversary stood as if transfixed. With sudden inward misgiving, I finished and pushed the coppers into the boatman's hand. Shaking his head and muttering to himself, he walked away; the ferry moved into midstream, and the crowd gradually returned to normal chatter.

As we neared the other shore, a Chinese gentleman made his way to my side and in excellent English asked, "Beg pardon, aren't you Doctor Basil?"

After an introduction—he was Chungking manager for one of the largest European firms in the Orient—there was the usual exchange of courtesies and small talk that always precedes business in any Chinese conversation. Finally my new acquaintance, who seemed a most likable person, came to the point. "Doctor, you've been here less than a year, haven't you?"

"Yes."

"Strange!" he murmured, as if thinking aloud.

"What's strange?"

"Your—" he hesitated somewhat apologetically—"your unusual vocabulary. I hope you don't mind my asking, but did you realize all that you said to this boatman?"

"I know what I started to say, though toward the end I surprised myself. What was the matter—were the tones mixed up?"

Amusement twitched at his lips. Suddenly he burst into laughter. "No, there was nothing wrong with your tones, Doctor; nobody could have failed to understand you. The trouble was with the expressions themselves. I keep wondering where you learned so many."

"You mean you wouldn't have used them?"

"I? Oh, no!" For a second he looked horrified, then humor again seized him. "You cursed that boatman from ancestors to posterity, until there was nothing left to be said. No coolie could have done it more fluently."

In the remaining minute or two before landing, we discussed the relative difficulties of learning English and Chinese. At parting, I told him that while my future language study might be limited to more ortho-dox sources, I had no intention of forgetting what had already been learned, since I'd seen for myself how effectively this could be used.

Afterwards, whenever I met him at Chungking civic affairs, he would ask with a twinkle in his eye, "Doctor, have you added anything exciting to your vocabulary lately?"

"Not a thing," was my usual retort. "It's becoming anemic from respectability."

However difficult, the language was simple enough compared with other problems. On return from the Southwest I had sent back my friend Lin's garments, with a note assuring him that they had been invaluable. He replied with a friendly line of acknowledgment, but I did not see him in person until a civic meeting occurred. A glance told me that he was worse, and after a warm exchange of greetings, I reminded, "It's time you stopped at the office."

Before he could comment on this, someone interrupted us and we found no other opportunity that day for private conversation. When the next week passed without his calling, my personal concern overcame professional policy, and I sent a chit to his business address, reiterating his need of an examination. Astonishingly the answer to this came from Lin's father; in it he stated his belief that I had already done everything possible for his son and that my further services would not be required. For the moment I felt as if I had been struck a physical blow; then, with the worst smart over, I tried to push both friendship and concern out of my mind.

Several times after that I ran into Lin at public affairs. We exchanged the usual conventional expressions, while fully conscious of a barrier of restraint. Then abruptly he dropped out of public life. There were rumors that his parents had sent to Hankow for two noted Chinese physicians to care for this son, and that these gentlemen were even now in command. Had another of Chungking's foreign doctors been called, I could have stopped worrying; as it was, I felt that my friend's fate was sealed.

At Christmas a package came from Lin, himself, containing rare gifts, and the note accompanying these was couched in such sincerity that acceptance seemed unavoidable. Later I was glad that pride had not been permitted to dictate their return.

Early in February a note from the sick man's younger brother asked me to call at their home the following afternoon. On arrival I was ushered into a room so crowded by members of the household that at first I could not find Lin himself. When, after endless introductions, I could turn attention to the patient, the sight of his pitiable, bloated body shocked me unspeakably. For the moment, caught offguard, I blurted out, "Why didn't you send for me before this, Lin?"

"It is good to have you come now," he answered; then for the benefit of his listening family, added in Chinese, "My good parents have spent much thought and strength on my welfare, but my body is stubborn and does not improve. For that reason they invite you here, *Beh Ih-seng*, to ask advice."

Yes, I thought silently, they call on the foreigner only when it is too late, for his weak, thready pulse had already revealed the worst. Seething inwardly over this needless sacrifice, I managed to murmur polite thanks for the honor, then turned again to the patient himself.

Lin interrupted my painful thoughts. "Your eyes tell me the truth of what I have felt for days—I am past being helped."

"Nonsense!" I contradicted, "I haven't even begun to work. First we'll see to diet." Pulling out a pad, I began jotting down food items.

When I looked up again, he resumed in English, "As I was taught in youth, I have tried always to observe the Five Relationships." (These fundamentals of Chinese society rest on mutual respect and consideration between emperor and subject; father and son; husband and wife; elder brother and younger brother; and friend with friend.) "Lately for good reasons, I have seemed to neglect the last of these, and that must have been difficult for you to understand. You will have to believe me when I say that there was no other way."

"If I had doubts, Lin, seeing you again has settled them."

"Good!" He lay back on his bed, then after a moment or two he continued slowly, as if weighing each word, "The Wheel of Life turns curiously for men. You are a foreigner and young; I am Chinese and middle-aged; yet we have been strangely drawn into intimacy."

"Rest and save your strength," I told him gently. "You and I do not need words to explain our friendship." For a quarter of an hour I sat there asking him questions about his condition; then in response to his request, recounted some of the amusing experiences in my trip to the Southwest. Conscious of his weariness, I asked suddenly, "Do you have any of the medicine I gave you?"

"Enough," he replied with a disturbingly prescient look.

"Have someone give you a dose at once; make them follow this diet list to the letter, and expect me first thing in the morning!"

As I rose to go, he spoke again in Chinese, asking his family to remember our personal relationship, if ever I needed help in Chungking.

"I am most unworthy of all these favors," I protested in the same tongue to the anxious group about us. "One thing only I wish—that you will do for my patient exactly as I have ordered."

However discouraging the case, each man has a fighting chance as long as he still breathes, and I racked my brain on the way home searching for some other medical weapon with which to fight Lin's disease. Two or three times daily I stopped in to see him, hoping against hope on each visit for an encouraging sign, but there were none, and by the end of the week he was dead.

Submerged in a mental slough those days that followed, I went about regular routine, freshly aware of the doctor's inability to work miracles, and saddened by personal loss. Even today with the crowded years between me and that time, I remember with a touch of wonder the rare quality of that relationship, which so completely broke down the barriers of age and creed and race.

Lin's death brought his younger brother and me into unexpected intimacy. Curious to learn why the dead man's illness had progressed so fast, I questioned him about the methods used by the Hankow doctors. Their theory and treatment follow: Food and drink enter the body through the stomach. There beneficent spirits pick it up and, by way of the blood stream, carry it to the heart. The heart separates good from harmful, distributing the first throughout the body and destroying the second in a central furnace, which is the source of body heat. In this furnace high temperature converts fluids into steam, and pressure forces this steam out. Some of it escapes as sweat through pores; but the most, chilled and condensed to water, passes by various internal canals into the bladder and is there discharged.

In this particular patient's case, it was explained, some unfriendly influence had interfered with the regular processes, and the steam, failing to condense, forced itself into the wrong channels and puffed up the limbs, dropsically. To correct this condition, the patient was made to drink an enormous quantity of liquid, which was depended upon to bring the condensation process back to normal and again fill the canals leading to the bladder. That the heart and other machinery of the body might be stimulated to greatest possible effort in this direction, a heavy diet of meat and highly seasoned sauces was prescribed. And the patient died.

Fantastic as this whole account may seem, their theory of elimination even though interpreted differently, was practically the same as our own, and the diagnosis and treatment of Lin's case presents a typical example, I think, of similarities and contrasts in Chinese and Western medicine. Through the long centuries the Chinese, lacking the mechanical and scientific devices that are Occidental therapy's common tools, have discovered an amazing number of truths about human anatomy. Many of these theories, far in advance of European medical knowledge at the time, were much more acceptable to modern medicine in their original form than they are today.

In the West profiteering corporations frequently capitalize enormously on the latest findings of research workers, who are themselves intent only on alleviating human suffering; so in China, charlatans seized these medical contributions of scholarly minds and adapted them to their own purposes.

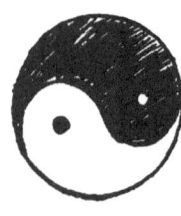

Permeating all Chinese beliefs and creeds was the old animistic religion that bestowed a spirit on each and every element of nature: sky, wind, rain, thunder, earth, rivers, trees, plants, animals, and man. The spirit of man was composed of a positive and a negative influence called Yang and Yin. Yang was the male principle—active, creative, progressive, its symbols the heavens, sun, light, warmth, youth, and strength. Yin, the female, was passive and, at the same time, destructive, symbolized by earth, moon, shade, winter, cold, old age, and weakness. The action of each of these on the other explained the diversities in human beings and influenced individual fates and fortunes.

In ancient China, this animism held to a rather high spiritual level, but after the sixth century B.C., Taoism, which like many other Oriental religions started out edifyingly well only to degenerate in time, became so thoroughly confused with the old, primitive faith that the great mass of people soon had nothing more than an accumulation of superstitions and fears in which to believe. For the educated, the austere tenets of Confucianism served as a stronghold against the popular theories of demonology, but even some of the enlightened were not always sure where they stood on the subject.

Medical practice, of course, offered a golden opportunity for playing on the fears of the ignorant man. *Feng-shui* literally "wind-water," and more broadly "the good and evil spirits carried on these" now complicated every theory. This lent an air of mystery to the simplest healing effort and, incidentally, provided an escape from blame when the practitioner made mistakes.

The Chinese treatment of tuberculosis offered what I considered an excellent example of superstition's influence on sound theory. It was clear that Chinese medicine had early recognized this disease as infectious, for their first step in treatment was to isolate the patient exactly as we do in the West. So far, good! But here the *Feng-shui* stepped in and proceeded to defeat what must have been the original idea, by placing the sick person in a dark, airless room. This removed him from the potent effects of Sun and Moon, considered dangerous in large amounts even to strong people and much more so to the weak.

Then, in direct contrast to the usual Chinese policy of overfeeding the ill, the tuberculous patient was permitted only a minimum diet. In this particular disease, it was explained, the evil spirits causing the disease lived off the body's food and could be expected to depart only when the supply of edibles was unsatisfactory.

To make up for this lack, the patient was given a special preparation containing nutritive and curative properties. This was supposed to be highly distasteful to the parasitic boarders; that it must have been even more unpalatable to the sick person seems not to have been considered.

The stomach was removed from a freshly killed hog, cleaned, then stuffed with the following ingredients: (1) a small portion of mud from ground at the north side of a sacred temple. (The north wind is supposed to have a purifying effect on earth exposed to it.); (2) a bunch of grass growing in a spot untouched by sunlight. (Here, again, is the avoidance of the Yang principle.); (3) a small, live terrapin; (4) a live toad; (5) trimmings from one set of finger nails excluding the little fingers. (This finger is considered the scholar's finger, and is accordingly respected.); (6) several hairs; (7) a handful of ashes from "idol paper" (imitation silver money used in sacrifices) burned in a temple urn; (8) tea made from a ginseng root.

After being stuffed, the stomach-bladder was steamed over an iron kettle for several hours.

On first reading, this horrible concoction sounds as if it might have been lifted from the pages of *Macbeth*, but there were some sound therapeutic elements contained in it. From the mud were obtained silicate and other minerals; from the grass, vitamins; from the terrapin, protein; from the toad, bufagin, a powerful heart stimulant; from the finger nails, calcium; from the ashes, charcoal. The ginseng was a demulcent; and the stomach, undergoing osmosis and dialysis, made its own contributions. Ginseng, the drug in which I had least faith, the Chinese had the most. No one of the other things in this prescription, except the terrapin with iodine content usually believed bad for tuberculous patients, could have been considered harmful aside from the fastidious or esthetic viewpoint. How many centuries this dose had been used, I have no idea, but foreign discovery of the value of bufagin and, in particular, of pig's stomach is of course quite recent.

Also, before we permit our nervous systems to react too unfavorably to the preparation, it is well to remember that only a generation or so ago, similar outlandish mixtures were common all over Europe and America, as they are in isolated sections today. Even in modern society, a good many "home remedies" are startling, to say the least. At present, with an intensive background, however brief, of sanitation and hygiene, we are apt to be unpleasantly affected by even the thought of such practices.

Doctors used to sights and smells grow callous, but on one occasion in Chungking, I found my own stomach reactions as queasy as those of any student nurse on her first appearance in surgery. A wealthy business man whose first wife had borne him only daughters, took a second consort, and during her first pregnancy sent for me. About sixteen years old, the girl was a victim of active pulmonary tuberculosis. I put her on a strict medical regimen and managed to carry her along to the seventh month, when the strain of a hemorrhage forced a premature birth.

The infant, weighing only a pound and one half, had the dark, wrinkled appearance of a tiny, ancient, wizened monkey. However, it was a boy and still alive, and the father was delighted. I found it difficult to make him understand that there was small foundation on which to base hope for its future. As far as he was concerned, the child had come into the world alive, and he was determined that here it should remain. For that matter so was I. I had an incubator constructed; placed one of our nurses in charge; and arranged to go with the father to the *lai ma* (wet nurse) market.

In the meantime a midwife had been taking care of the mother, and I now turned my attention to that quarter. As was customary with Chinese women, the girl's hair was sleeked back; and high on either temple a large pinfeather from a rooster's tail had been drilled through the skin to the bone. These were for the purpose of making holes through which the evil spirit, the cause of the premature birth, might leave the body.

While I watched, the old woman half filled a cup with water. In it she placed a clot of blood from the discarded placenta, and after stirring this with her dirty fingers, gave it to the young mother to drink. At this point, I felt that I, as well as mother and child, needed medical attention, and for a number of hours

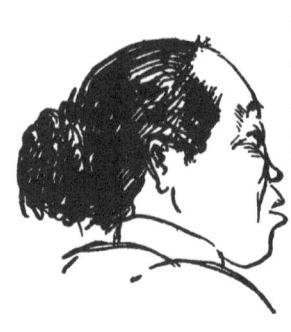

afterward, I had little appetite for food. When I ventured to protest this treatment, the midwife gave me clearly to understand that she would brook no interference in her job. On this point the father agreed, insisting that my full attention be given to his son, and we started off on our errand.

At the *lai ma* market we found about a dozen women available for service. Few Chinese mothers who can afford wet nurses feed their own infants, and women of the lowest classes who have babies of their own hire out for this purpose. I selected two for this child and took them over to the hospital for physical examination. Satisfied about health, I next had them soaked in baths of soap and lysol suds, and their breasts scrubbed, all of this much to their horror. These two, under supervision of hospital nurses, now took turns supplying the milk, by means of a Breck feeder (an oversized medicine dropper attached to a bulb syringe) to the child in the incubator.

Due to underweight, abscesses formed beneath the end of the baby's spine, but these were drained, and he seemed none the worse for wear. By eight months he weighed five pounds and was quite alert mentally.

Shortly after that I had to be away, and during my absence, Chinese doctors were called in by the Number One wife, for the boy's mother had died soon after birth. Under their treatment the infant became worse daily. To quiet its irritable crying, opium smoke was

12

blown into the baby's mouth. This provoked a bad reaction in his congenitally weak lungs, and before long he was dead.

Up to this time the father had spent silver lavishly on the care of his son. Now that the child could no longer perpetuate the family name, or pay respects to ancestral tablets, he was put in a cheap little box and buried without any ceremony whatever. Such a course of action seems callous indeed to the average Westerner, but the Chinese is above all things a realist. What's done is done—*Muh iu fa tz!*

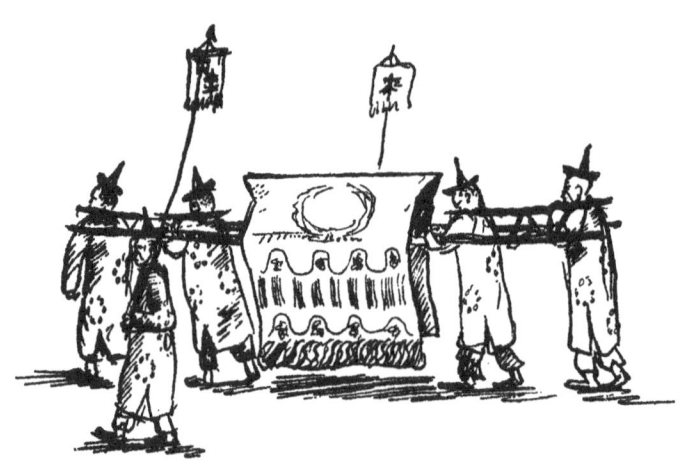

CHAPTER XI

"Only the Wealthy Can Afford to Visit the Law Courts" (*Proverb*)

It seems hardly necessary for me to discuss at length the well-known virtues of Chinese servants. The average servant on entering one's employ promises that the safety of everything under the roof will be "on his body," and he will risk much personally to keep his word. Loyalty is one of the strongest of Chinese characteristics, and in trouble particularly, this quality comes to the fore.

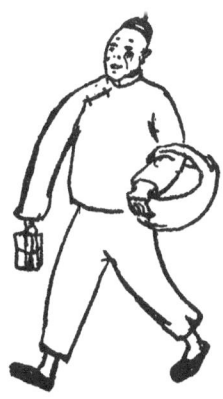

He is willing and indefatigable, working seven days in the week from dawn until late at night, this last hour depending upon the habits of his employer. Extra guests are his delight, since these add gaiety and mild excitement to the ordinary, dull routine.

When a mistress, an hour before a meal, informs her cook that there will be five or six more people at table than were expected, he merely remarks philosophically, *"Ko ee tien ih dien shui!"* (Can add a little water—with the basic word, *soup*, understood.) After this, he hustles the coolie and table boy to neighboring homes and borrows for the occasion whatever delicacies may be in those larders. That the neighbors will not receive the special dishes their respective cooks had promised them bothers him not at all; never shall his household lose face by providing poorly for visitors—not if he can in any way prevent this calamity.

To balance so many virtues, most Chinese servants have two faults: they are careless about cleanliness, and they will struggle unceasingly to do things after their own fashion rather than that of the employer. For the foreigner in China the servant problem is usually limited to the two difficulties mentioned. Maud and I proved to be the exceptions to this pleasant rule, and as a result, had a most unhappy and expensive experience.

One chilly morning after hospital rounds, I stopped in at our residence to pick up a coat and hat before making city calls. Neither was in its accustomed place, and when search and servant questioning failed to recover the missing garments, as well as a number of others from my wardrobe, I sent for the police. Any old China hand reading this will at once smile at the foolishness of this step, for the field of criminal law offers no common meeting ground to foreigner and Chinese.

In response to my appeal there appeared an officer with a bodyguard. After a great deal of talking about the affair, this worthy left to reappear on the morrow with the Police Commissioner and *his* bodyguard.

"*Beh Ih-seng* is certain the garments have been stolen, *hsi puh hsi?*" asked the Commissioner gravely.

"Positive!"

"They are not in the house?"

"Certainly not!"

"Better that we too search the house before accusing anyone!"

I agreed at once, not realizing that the process would require two days and a search of all neighboring buildings as well as our own residence. When this effort, as I had expected, proved fruitless, the Commissioner announced sadly, "We must take all of your servants to prison."

Our staff protested volubly, demanding rights as Guild members to a hearing with the Servants' Guild Committee. This petition was granted, and on the following day twenty-five people, or more, met in our yard to hold temporary court. The cook, as chief servant, came first in the list of suspects but was disposed of immediately. Since he was the Number One worker, he represented authority in the domicile and, if held responsible for misdemeanor, would automatically involve all below him in rank. Finally the coolie (the one servant of whose innocence Maud and I were certain) belonging at the bottom of the scale in Guild groups and accordingly incapable of dragging anyone down with him, was made the scapegoat, arrested, and taken to the *yamen* (official court). The other servants were

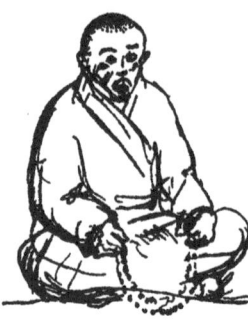

held on a parole that required daily reporting to the Guild but did not permit them to work. However, that they might use every opportunity to clear their reputations by further investigations on the premises, the authorities gave them the freedom of our compound.

One day the cook and table-boy, accompanied by a priest and a crowd of hangers-on, appeared in the front yard and proceeded to conduct a divining ceremony for the purpose of establishing guilt. A fire was made on a bare spot of earth, and after a long incantation had been said over this, two chickens were brought forward for sacrifice. These were dismembered, piece by piece, with the priest and table-boy (the servant we suspected of the theft) officiating in fine style; and as the sections burned, prayers were offered for the recovery of my garments. From time to time some one of the hangers-on would come forward and suggest that I send to such and such a place on such and such a street, since it seemed likely my clothes had strayed there. This ceremony undoubtedly offered an opening for the guilty to reveal the truth without loss of face, so I followed several leads. But no clothes were found then or later, and for some time I was forced to amuse the Chungking public by appearing in a variety of ill-fitting garments lent by generous friends.

Several weeks later a message from the *yamen* requested my appearance there. On arrival I found our old coolie, Lao Hsiu, in a dark and clammy dungeon below street level. The sole furniture in the narrow space was a bench on which he sat, slept, and ate his one daily meal—a bowl of rice.

Already he looked half dead, but with a coolie's usual ability to endure hardship, he made little complaint about personal wretchedness. His entire conversation was limited to asserting his innocence. I told him that both Mrs. Basil and I had complete faith in him, and a little later I asked the *yamen* official for the poor fellow's immediate release.

After a great deal of palaver they agreed, on condition that I pay Lao Hsiu's board bill while there—a sum of forty-five dollars (Mexican). There was nothing to do but accept these terms, not only to remedy injustice but also because I was afraid the coolie might die in that hole—a burden of responsibility which Law and Tradition would lay on my shoulders.

When Lao Hsiu and I reached home, the news of his release had already preceded us. A representative of the Guild came to greet me with the word that the coolie might not again enter my employ. Under my roof, it was claimed, he had been arrested on a charge of theft; to remain there after that would rob him of face entirely.

I turned to Lao Hsiu. "Do you wish to work for us?" I asked.

"Of course, *Beh Ih-seng*, but the Guild will not permit me to break custom. Only evil to both of us will come of it."

It was quite clear by this time that the victim of a theft—not the thief—paid dearly for the offense. I had lost my clothes, forty-five dollars, and a good coolie; and the whole compound had been turned into a public meeting place for political riffraff.

Suddenly the worm turned. I told the table-boy without further ado that I was through with him, and he would have to hunt another job.

"The Guild must decide that, *Beh Ih-seng!* If you dismiss me, I shall have no face."

"Suit yourself," I replied. "If you stay on, you'll have no face, either. You have never been a very good table-boy, and now that we have lost our coolie, you will have to do his work in the future."

As I had expected, this unheard-of demotion turned the trick, and he promptly resigned. Surprisingly enough, petty thieving of canned goods and other small objects continued after his dismissal, and we were at a loss how to account for it.

One morning the faithful Lao Hsiu sought me out. He seemed to have something burdening his mind, but at last I drew from him a warning against callers at hours when the *Si-mu* and I were not about the house. After the coolie's departure, I took this matter up with the gateman, who finally admitted that every afternoon when I was in the hospital and Maud was resting in her bedroom, a cousin of our former table-boy appeared, asked for me, and then hung around the house for an hour or so on the pretense of awaiting my arrival. This was all the information I wanted. When the cousin next came, I met him in person with the threat that if anybody from his family ever entered our compound again, I would lead him straight to the Tuchun of the Province. With that the matter was settled for all time, but it left me wary of all that had to do with Chinese courts.

I really should not have needed the personal experience to develop this attitude, for the foreign community had a long and discouraging list of lawsuits on record. Our own hospital was still paying dearly for one, concerning a delirious typhoid patient who, left alone for a moment, had jumped through a window and died. The woman's husband had promptly sued the hospital for negligence and, winning the case, had been paid. A year later her mother sued; the next, her father-in-law; and just before I left Chungking, her great-grandfather. We lost in each instance—tried as it was in a Chinese court prejudiced against foreign medicine—and this in spite of all that the American Consul could do as mediator.

The Woman's Hospital had been through even worse affairs. As its name implied, that institution did not ordinarily take men patients, but as in all the other hospitals, when the military demanded admission, they got it. On one occasion of this sort, a general had been ordered an enema. The student nurse who prepared and administered this, confused carbolic acid with the

solution prescribed, and fifteen minutes later the patient
died. In the excitement the nurse managed to flee from
the city, and the ensuing lawsuit named the hospital
management responsible for the mistake. An enormous
sum was paid the family, as well as generous rental to
the temple in which the coffin reposed awaiting a
burial date and location which astrologers considered
propitious. In this particular case interment was delayed
five years, and during that time the hospital continued
to pay temple rent.

Another case in the same hospital, of unusual interest
to all but the victimized establishment, came as a result
of an urgent call from a private house for the services
of a Chinese woman physician. When the doctor reached
the place and was ushered into a room in the women's
quarters, she could find no one among those present
who seemed in need of attention.

"Where is the patient?" she asked.

The others pointed to a young and unhappy-looking
woman sitting near the window. After a brief examination, the physician inquired, "Why do you think
this girl is sick?"

The oldest woman in the group, apparently the
matriarch of the establishment, answered with a surprised air, "Is it possible the doctor cannot see for
herself? This one, my eldest grandson's wife, is first
very hot, then very cold. She eats little, and her temper
fires at trifles."

The physician sat and studied the patient. The girl had neither temperature nor chills at the moment, but that she looked unhappy was certainly true. Chinese herself, the doctor wondered if there were more to this than that which showed on the surface. However, the other women present seemed genuinely concerned about the patient, and there was nothing else to do but suggest hospitalization for physical tests. A few hours later, the girl was admitted to the institution. She offered no protests about examinations, but remained stonily silent under questioning.

Late that afternoon her father-in-law called. The nurse, stepping courteously into the corridor, overheard the old man, who had evidently been looking around the place, say, "There is an unused well outside this window. I am afraid you may throw yourself in it."

When the attendant repeated this to the physician, she was told, "It may have no meaning. Also, to drown in the little water that seeps into that well would be difficult indeed; but tomorrow morning we'll move the patient to another room! Meanwhile, see that she is not left alone for one minute!"

At the following daybreak the patient asked for a bedpan, and her nurse, unable at the moment to find anyone else to go for the article, slipped down the hall to the bathroom where they were kept. When she returned a few minutes later, the patient was gone.

A brief search discovered the missing girl already drowned, head downward in the foot or two of water in the well.

Notified of her death, the father-in-law, accompanied by eight soldiers, stormed into the hospital demanding that the Chinese doctor and the night nurse who had been on duty appear with them at once before a Court of Law. These agreed willingly enough, only to find that the father-in-law was a judge and that the case had been moved from the hospital district to his court in another section of the city. There, the following charges were laid against them: 1. The hospital was negligent in leaving windows open at night when, as everyone knew, windows should be closed after dark for the sake of health as well as for safety. 2. The nurse on duty must have slept while the woman was dying, and then, fearful of responsibility, had probably pushed the body out of the window into the well and called it a suicide.

A long period of questioning followed, but nothing was settled. Three times a week for several months, doctor and nurse were required to appear in that court for the purpose of rehashing the affair from beginning to end.

One day they failed to return, and when word reached the hospital that the doctor had been imprisoned on a charge of manslaughter, the foreign nurse-superintendent took things into her own hands.

Dismissing all convalescents and transferring the very ill to other institutions, she closed the building, arranged for a foreign bondsman, and went down to the prison. Gaining permission to see the Chinese doctor in her cell, the foreigner then refused to leave, insisting that as superintendent she was as much involved as the doctor and the two of them would have to be imprisoned and tried together.

This presented complications, for an American, under extraterritorial rights, could not be imprisoned in a Chinese *yamen*. When all attempts to make her leave failed—the guards did not dare to try the use of physical force with a foreigner—both were released. This, however, was merely a reprieve, for the father-in-law judge had now lost face and was ready for further vengeance. To escape, the Chinese doctor hastily decided on a vacation down river. She managed to elude soldiers at the gate by going over the City Wall at night and then descending to the shore of the Little River, was carried by sampan to a French steamer anchored in the Yangtze.

For almost a year the hospital remained closed. Civic indignation works slowly in China, as elsewhere, but finally a delegation of Chungking citizens begged that the institution be reopened. This plea was granted by the Mission only when the Chungkingese themselves forced the father-in-law to sign the petition, and thus put an end to the quarrel.

What lent this incident a macabre interest was its motivation, eventually uncovered. The dead girl had been compelled to put up with criminal advances from her natural protector while her husband was away studying near the coast. Desperate over the situation, she had twice tried to commit suicide. The old villain in the case realized that if she succeeded in doing this under his roof, her family in another town would demand explanation and justice. To avoid this, he had decided on the hospital as an acceptable place for her demise, and so the affair had been carried out.

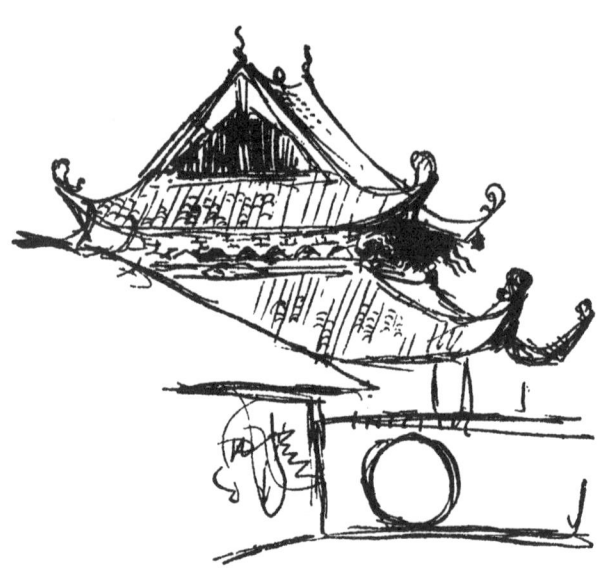

CHAPTER XII

"An Opium Den Is a Lamp on the Road to Death"
(Proverb)

Perhaps the chief reason for Szechuen's independent attitude throughout history lay in the ability of the province to sustain itself. The soil was unbelievably rich and fertile, and there was almost no crop that would not flourish. Sugar, tobacco, and many important herbs and native drugs, as well as the more common foodstuffs, grew in these fields. Great salt wells, together with groves of tung oil, insect wax, and lacquer trees, brought in rich revenue from the outside world.

Silkworms were of an unusually hardy breed, making West China crepe and pongee as fine and durable silks as the world can produce. The hills were rich in minerals, and traveling about the countryside, one often came across small coal mines hand-operated by men and boys.

To the stream of local products that flowed through Chungking's water gates toward the outer world was added those of Eastern Tibet, Northern Kweichow, and Yunnan. Hides, bristles, tea, rice, drugs, straw-braid, silks, and wool packed the holds of steamers

179

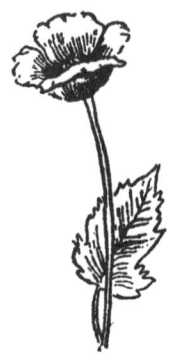

and junks bound for Hankow, where most of the shipments were redistributed.

But if everything else seemed to thrive in Szechuen soil, so did the poppy. In the early half of the nineteenth century when Indian opium was first forced in quantity on the China market, the supplies traveled the perilous overland route from Southern Asia to Chungking; then were shipped down river from there. It took the Szechuen warlords a very short time to discover that they could produce the drug in unlimited quantity locally, and greatly undersell its import price. Put into immediate practice, this plan paid better than in the promoters' greediest dreams, and fortunes were amassed overnight.

The Empress Dowager, determined to nip the evil in the bud, now stopped all local production of opium by exacting the death penalty for growing it. This severe program achieved remarkable results, but in the chaotic years following the Revolution, when the Manchu Empress and her dynasty were overthrown, the poppy began to flourish once more.

During my residence in Chungking, I met the drug and its evil results on every hand. In 1931 alone, the China *Year Book* estimated the Szechuen export of opium at 21,000,000 ounces. Most farmers, begrudging every inch of soil taken from food-producing, hated the very sight of the slender, graceful plants. But they were helpless to remedy the situation. As the Imperial

Edict had once inflicted the death sentence on owners
of poppy fields, now it became equally dangerous for a
man not to plant. When nonproducers were not more
severely punished, they were forced to pay a "lazy
tax" on land that grew no opium.

With the price running from sixty cents to more than
two dollars (Mexican) an ounce, there was naturally
an enormous amount of smuggling done. The foreign
captains on the Upper River steamers considered this
contraband traffic one of their chief problems. Searching for it was like hunting the proverbial needle in a
haystack, for the opium was often hidden in the most
minute quantities and in such unlikely places as can-
vas seams or the bindings on deck mats. A traveler's
fan or umbrella might carry the drug in its handle;
his innocent-looking spectacle case might hold a good
deal more. The nose was the best of all detection
agencies, for no matter how carefully the drug was
wrapped, its sickeningly sweet odor was bound to seep
out.

Unsatisfied with the revenue from exporting opium,
the politicians licensed dens in every available town
and city. Chungking had several thousand such places
when I was there, and all too frequently we were asked
to attend victims of an overdose.

One Sunday morning I received an urgent call from
a wealthy home over in Kiang-beh. I had been in
Chungking just about a year at the time, and my

13

language was still limited. The household in question was new to my acquaintance, and with strangers the foreign student of the language had much more difficulty in making himself understood than with his Chinese intimates. Tradespeople, hospital attendants, and most of the officials were accustomed to listening carefully when a Westerner spoke the native tongue, exactly as we do in trying to understand a transplanted European's English. This was not true, however, of those citizens who lacked intimate contacts with foreigners. Many among them worked on the assumption that we were not mentally equipped to learn Chinese, and therefore they did not recognize their own speech when we used it.

Since opium cases often had unpleasant complications, I suggested that Doctor Tu accompany me to make sure that there should be no misunderstanding between patient, family, and myself with regard to methods. Tu had gone through a number of affairs with me, and I had grown to like him greatly. He was an unusually tall and good-looking Northern Chinese, with plenty of initiative and skill. At the hospital he was Resident in Surgery, and I never had to question the integrity of his work.

We ferried across the Lin in a sampan, and soon reached our destination, an imposing residence of many wings. The patient was, surprisingly enough, the patriarch of the establishment. A confirmed opium user, he had been increasing his daily amounts until the family became frightened and curtailed the supply. Desperate for habitual dosage, the old man had resorted to the well-known method of scraping the poisonous residue from his pipe and drinking this in a cup of wine.

I had treated a number of similar cases with a stomach pump and sometimes revived them, but this one had done the job so thoroughly that I found him already in a dying condition. I had Tu repeat my explanation that the case was past helping so that there might be no doubts left in their minds.

This word left them panic-stricken. The powerful and inescapable sense of filial duty now convinced them that by interfering with their Elder's habits, they had killed him. They begged to know what I usually did in such cases. I explained the use of a stomach pump, and they seized on this as a last hope.

I objected. "Tu, make it clear to them that swallowing a stomach tube often strangles strong people. With this old man already gasping, he may die even as we insert it."

Doctor Tu stressed carefully what I had said, so that there was no possibility of misunderstanding, but still they insisted that the foreign way be tried.

Against my better judgment I agreed. The tube was inserted, and the pumping continued until all odor of opium was gone from the waste.

Then when I removed the apparatus, the patient, as I had momentarily expected, breathed his last. At once the whole household seemed to go crazy and, as I had also expected, declared that the pumping had been the direct cause of death.

For an interminable period Doctor Tu and I argued the case with them; then recognizing a stalemate, decided to leave. We were informed that the local officials had been sent for and that, while Doctor Tu was free to leave, I should have to remain on the spot until a thorough and satisfactory investigation had been made concerning the cause of this death.

This being my second experience at involuntary detention, I sat down with the idea of being thoroughly uncomfortable for an indefinite period. Although their intentions toward me might be dubious, my hosts had no idea of neglecting the demands of hospitality, for a servant now appeared with bowls of tea. Doctor Tu accepted his with exaggerated politeness. I refused mine.

I was beginning to worry about the hospital's routine for this day. Since Chinese affairs always move slowly, I might be held over here for twenty-four hours or more, and it seemed advisable for Tu to return and help the other interne, Wei, cover our rounds. When I put this into speech, Tu demurred.

"I don't like this affair, Doctor," he said in an undertone of English, between sips of tea. "If it becomes known that they cut down the amount of opium the old man had been using, thereby forcing him to eat the residue, which everybody knows is poison, public opinion will ruin their name. Someone must be blamed for their mistake; and Fortune has given you into their hands."

"If I knew these Kiang-beh officials, it might help!"

Tu nodded. "Yes; but as it is, *Beh Ih-seng*, they are not likely to risk offending a wealthy family for the sake of a foreigner."

"Well, they can't throw me into the *yamen* without becoming involved with the higher-ups."

Deviltry flickered in Tu's eye. "At the moment the *yamen* might be the safest place to be."

I considered this thoughtfully. "No, I think one place is as safe as another. I have a hunch that for me personally this affair is not going to amount to much more than a lot of inconvenience. What does concern me is the hospital. Although they don't need money, they may sue just for the sake of proving the case in their favor." The possibility of a lawsuit was the one fear that dogged my steps the whole time I was in Chungking. "You go on back as I suggested and send off the note I'm going to write."

I had just had an idea. Hastily I scribbled a line to the Captain of the Navy gunboat, describing my predicament, and asking him to look into the matter if I were not released within twenty-four hours.

Tu was meanwhile writing something of his own. With the two notes in his hand he said, "If you don't mind, *Beh Ih-seng*, I will stay here and send these by one of their coolies. I think it will be better."

When I agreed, he asked for a servant to carry a note to the hospital. When the man arrived, Tu pushed the notes and some money into his hand, and after what seemed a lengthy explanation, sent him on his way.

A few minutes later the gateman knocked on the door and asked to speak to the oldest man present, who was evidently the dead patriarch's immediate successor.

This worthy listened carefully to the message, then dismissing the man, came back to face me with a disturbed expression. "Why did *Beh Ih-seng* write to the warship?" he asked uncertainly.

Discovering this to be the cause of his worry, I made the most of it. "It is custom!" I replied in the stock Chinese phrase. "You, Sir, sent for your officials; I sent for mine also. They can consider this matter together."

"But *Beh Ih-seng* himself can talk with our officials."

"Never! In our country a prisoner always has a representative speak for him."

His eyebrows took the elevator upward. "But *Beh Ih-seng* is not a prisoner!"

"I am not permitted to leave."

"Truly all under this roof are miserable, stupid creatures. This is a misunderstanding, indeed. *Beh Ih-seng* may leave when he wishes."

I remained seated. "If you will permit me, Sir, I shall remain until your officials arrive. As long as you think I caused the death of your honorable parent, I am most unhappy."

"Lay down your heart, Doctor. It was not you, but that hospital instrument."

"But I, not the hospital, used it. That is what I wish my government representative to help yours understand."

Meanwhile Tu had accepted more boiling water for his tea leaves and was quietly enjoying the second bowl. Our host directed the next sentence to him, and after a moment Tu informed me that they would be very happy to explain to their officials that neither I nor the hospital was in any way to blame for this trouble.

My brows set in a deep frown as I pretended to think this over carefully. It was all too clear that they were growing more nervous every moment. Their officials might arrive at any time and find to their personal indignation a squashed case. Still more terrifying was the thought of seeing the American gunboat steam into position before Kiang-beh and begin to shell the town. Then this household would be in hot water not only with a foreign government but with

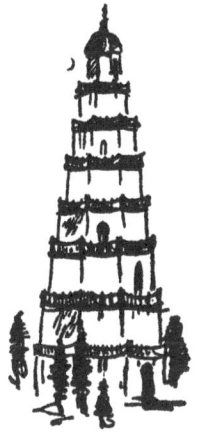

their own town as well. In this suddenly complicated situation they were experiencing the truth of a familiar proverb, "He who catches a hedgehog has difficulty letting it go."

When I spoke, it was with deliberation. "If, Sir, you wish to write down that you do not hold us responsible, I shall be most grateful."

"At once, Doctor. And what do we owe for your excellent services?"

"Twenty-five dollars (Mexican) for the trip to Kiang-beh; twenty-five more for the extra hours spent under this roof."

Until now the others in the room had been as silent as the dead. These figures made them come to life. There were murmured objections from all quarters. I could see them thinking: "*Ai-ya*, this is too much! This foreigner not only refuses to sacrifice himself, but he charges us double the usual fee."

The elder now proposed, "Tomorrow we can carry the silver to the hospital for *Beh Ih-seng*."

I sat down again. In households like this there was always a supply of money on hand. "If you wish a little time for finding the silver, I shall be glad to wait," I suggested mildly.

Within ten minutes, Tu and I, in possession of fifty dollars and a signed paper absolving us and the hospital of complicity in this death, made our way through the ornately lacquered gateway.

"It was lucky for us that chit-coolie was talkative. I supposed that if we let them know a note was going to the gunboat, they would seize it."

Tu smiled. "They didn't get the chance. I paid him three hundred cash (about twenty cents Mexican) to wag his tongue at the right moment."

I stared completely puzzled.

Doctor Tu went on with relish, "I suggested that as he went through the gatehouse, he could make all the servants, hanging around, jealous by telling them he was about to board the American gunboat."

"Well, it certainly worked," I said admiringly. "What they didn't guess was that the note asked 'Navy' to look me up after twenty-four hours, not before." I lighted a cigarette, then added, "You have certainly helped me out of a lot of difficulties, since I arrived, Tu."

"Life used to be so much duller," he murmured to the air about him.

When we reached the hospital, the other interne who had received Tu's note and was trying to make all our rounds, stopped to bombard us with questions.

While Tu explained, I slipped into my office and sent a note to the gunboat captain telling him all was well. When I finally reached home, Maud was coming out the gate on her way to the hospital. "What in the world does this mean?" she asked and held out a chit from "Navy" asking if I'd returned.

"Just a little mixup," I told her easily, "in which Tu did some quick thinking, and the hospital came off with an extra twenty-five dollars to the good."

"Grand! With what we've got toward that Women's Ward fund, this twenty-five dollars will buy all the cretonne needed to brighten the windows. I'll order it from Shanghai by the next mail."

In my mind I had already tried out the sum toward three other hospital purposes. Well, I thought, accepting Fortune as it came, I would not now have the trouble of making a choice.

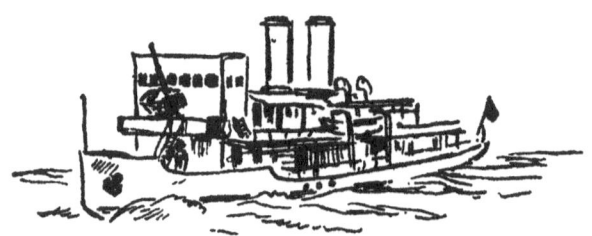

CHAPTER XIII

"Good Reason He Has to Be Sad!"

According to Mencius, "Three things are unfilial; the chief among these is to have no posterity."

Similar statements are to be found everywhere in Chinese learning, and the people, high and low, dutifully heed them to the letter. A man's hope of future existence lies in having a son who will bring his father's name to the attention of Heaven and Earth during family observance of ancestral rites. A woman has no such long-range interest; her peace and happiness in the immediate present depend on ability to produce sons.

Birth is the one subject of thought and speech in China that holds unflagging interest for all listeners. References to it are to be found in the most ordinary conversations, regardless of the speakers' ages. It is common knowledge that pregnant women often crave unusual items of food, so when a child asks for something salt or sour rather than a sweet, the customary exclamation is, "Are you about to bear a son?"

Since the greater part of a foreign doctor's effort in China must be devoted to obstetrics—ten to twenty times as much as a general practitioner's at home—I found myself collecting a mass of odd tales and super-stitions about maternity. One of the best known Chinese volumes is *Kuang Hsu Chuan Hsu* (*Complete Book on How To Obtain Children*), and the people quote from this on all occasions.

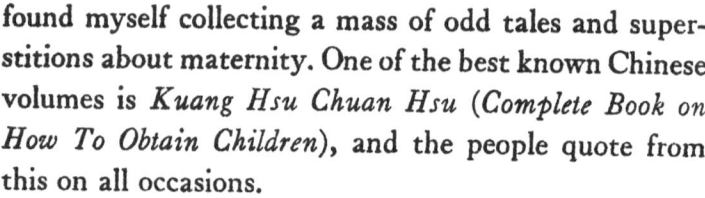

Since daughters are destined to marry early and become members of other families, sons are naturally of first importance, and sex determination before birth is a subject of interest to all. The most complicated method given is by arithmetical calculation: "Multiply seven times seven; add to this the number of months of pregnancy; subtract the age of the pregnant woman, and add nineteen." If the result is an odd number, the child will be a boy; if an even number, a girl."

This mathematical solution fails to take into account that the months of pregnancy would increase, while the mother's age in years would remain the same. When I asked a Chinese scholar about this, as well as the reasons for using the numbers seven and nineteen, his answer was uncertain. He seemed to think that this formula was a free translation from the ancient *Book of Changes*.

Another belief stated that if the embryo faces for-ward, thus enlarging the womb, or if the father should be older and stronger physically than the mother, the child will be a boy. On the other hand, if the mother suffers greatly from nausea during pregnancy, the off-spring is certain to be a girl.

Warnings about prenatal influences are legion. A pregnant woman must be very careful while preparing vegetables. Should the child's body move when the prospective mother is cutting a turnip in two, the turnip halves must be stuck together again at once—otherwise the child will arrive with a gash in its forehead. If the sun cast a shadow on the mother's face when she is peeling vegetables (I never learned why so much stress was laid on vegetables, though it is possible that some primitive analogy between the two forms of life was in mind), the child will be born with a harelip.

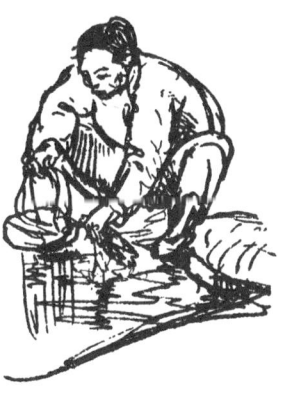

A Chinese woman who was unusually intelligent and discreet of speech told me in all seriousness that a cousin of hers, because of just such carelessness, had given birth to seven children with harelips. My first mental reaction to this was to wonder why the mother in the case had not paid someone else to peel vegetables, or at least to have learned, herself, to avoid shadows. My second was to question the probability of such an occurrence, though I had no slightest reason for doubting the veracity of the one who related the story. A harelip is caused by an abnormal distribution of tissue cells and is always a rarity. To consider seven of these cases in one family stretched medical credulity to the limit.

Dreams during pregnancy are supposed to contain all sorts of threats. I was told of one instance in which a woman, four months pregnant, woke moaning from an afternoon nap. "What is the matter?" demanded her sister in the same room.

There was no reply, and the prospective mother continued speechless for a full hour or more. When her child was born, it was totally deaf and, therefore, mute.

During pregnancy a Chinese woman is advised to avoid looking at a monkey, a tiger, or an actor wearing an ugly mask, for any one of these may leave an impression on the unborn child.

If these theories sound absurd in Western ears, it is only because man's protective instinct is to forget whenever possible his own close links with the primitive. No other profession is weighted so heavily by accumulated ignorance from the past as is Medicine, and, of all its branches, obstetrics is the most backward. The art of healing has always had to fight quackery, suspicion, and superstition. Where the important question of propagation has been concerned, these obstacles have been almost insurmountable.

Sometimes it was the physician who contributed the most harm to his cause. Over two thousand years ago Hippocrates made the cynical statement: "The patient must combat the disease along with the physician." Later Galen, commenting on this remark, adds: "The practice of certain physicians is like playing at the dice when what turns up may occasion the greatest mischief to their patients."

I found few beliefs in China for which America did not have parallels. More than one of my patients here at home has believed implicitly that attacks of heartburn during pregnancy are certain indications of the child's being a boy. Many more feel that bad dreams, ugly sights, and frightening experiences may mark a child for life. One of the commonest of these fears is that if the prospective mother sees a mouse run across the floor, the child will be disfigured by moles.

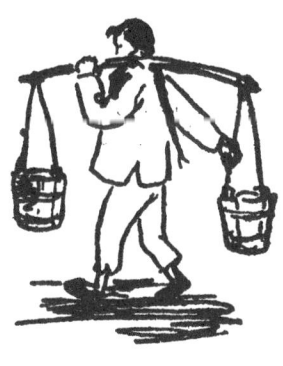

In preparation for childbirth, the average Chinese woman shows more common sense than do some of her Western sisters. Centuries have made the Eastern woman conscious, perhaps cruelly so, that her child, rather than herself, is the important factor in the family scheme of life. Even the well-to-do mothers are urged to increase physical exercise; the poor one continues most of her usual tasks in house and field, and both are warned against the dangers of stretching or lifting heavy objects.

Despite the importance centering around childbirth, abortion is practiced in China as everywhere else. Proportionately, these are fewer in number than in the West; this is true also of abnormal deliveries. The Chinese racial characteristics of small-headed infants is the chief reason for births without instruments or lacerations, and the result is that few women in China have carcinoma of the cervix. Seventy-five percent of my patients in Chungking were women; in my whole

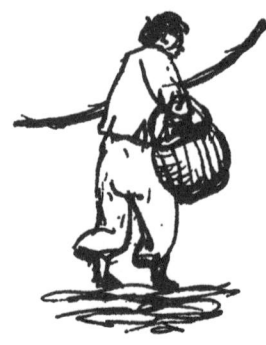

experience I did not find a half-dozen cases of this trouble.

What I did consider most remarkable was the amount of suffering and torment the young Chinese mother was able to endure at the hands of traditional midwifery. There seemed every reason for most of them to die of infections. A case of my own offered spectacular proof of one woman's physical resistance. A hurried delivery call had come to me from the other end of the city, and I arrived on the scene only to discover that the mother was already close to death in eclampsia. This was a new patient, and I asked the family bluntly why they had delayed sending for me until it was too late to be of service.

"We know the mother is the same as dead, Honorable Doctor; it is our hope that you will save the child."

A hasty examination had revealed that the baby was still alive. I decided now to wait until I felt absolutely certain the mother couldn't live, then I would take it from her. Equipped for an ordinary delivery, I had nothing with which to perform a Caesarian Section save a common scalpel. When the mother's gasps began to grow more tortured, I rubbed a little alcohol and ether on the site of operation and delivered a fine boy.

While I was examining him, the gasping suddenly ceased. For a split second I thought the woman was dead; then she drew several long, deep breaths. I hurried the baby into waiting arms, sent someone out to buy glucose on the street, and next injected heart stimulants into the patient. The wound was bleeding freely, and I let this continue, considering it the best way of avoiding infection and of carrying off the uremic poison. Before circulation became depleted, the incision was sutured and the woman given further hypodermics of glucose. She recovered completely— a fact that surprised no one so much as the doctor. Being familiar with Chinese delivery methods, the woman had undoubtedly been subjected to all sorts of strain and discomfort before my arrival, and personally, I had taken liberties far beyond those of accepted medical practice. At home these methods might have laid me open to the charge of malpractice, but in primitive fields of medicine one learns to use whatever may be at hand. Osler stressed the importance of common sense in emergencies rather than that of depending entirely on set rules and mechanical aids, and this was one instance when that policy seemed to work. In such freedom of action, though, there is the ever-present danger of growing careless and of taking unnecessary risks.

The New Year's festival, the most important in the Chinese calendar, often worked havoc with my delivery programs. Any number of taboos have accumulated through the ages in connection with this celebration. No Chinese will willingly mention pain, disease, or any other kind of trouble during that period, for fear of

14

future ill consequences. The home, where all the ancestral rites are being observed, assumes an even more hallowed position than usual in men's minds. The last thing that a sick member of the family wishes to do is to leave its sheltering roof. Birth, unfortunately, pays no attention to such creature whims or desires.

A patient for whom I had cared through the whole period of pregnancy reached her hour on New Year's Day. All arrangements had been made for hospital service, but the woman refused to leave home. When, in response to a much delayed message, I finally arrived there, a midwife had already delivered the hapless infant, in several sections. I looked at the small mangled body and noticed a tiny shoe filled with rice tied to one of its legs.

"For what purpose was this?" I asked curiously.

"This child was upside down, *Beh Ih-seng*," the old woman explained. "In a case like that, when a foot emerges, a shoe is attached to help the rest of the body walk out, and the rice is to give the child strength."

For the foreign woman in China, giving birth is, at best, a precarious business. Physically depleted by trying climate and frequently the victim of some tropical disease for which the foreigner has no established immunity, the pregnant American or European woman is often handicapped at the start. To these hazards is added such uncertainty of medical attention that many of the community women travel all the way to Shanghai for the culminating event.

In Chungking this uncertainty was due not to the lack of foreign physicians, for there were several, but rather to the size of the field. This included the city proper, its suburbs, Kiang-beh, and the Hills. Most of the foreign business people lived in the last location, and in order to reach them the Yangtze had to be crossed, a time-consuming trip with the further complications of limited hours for transportation. No boatman in his right mind would willingly brave that broad, dangerous current after dark. This meant that any Hills' case detaining me past sunset necessitated my remaining there overnight. But no matter how urgent city and hospital cases might be, if a prospective mother in The Hills sent word her hour had come, there was no alternative but to go directly to her.

When the wife of one of our friends in the oil business became pregnant for the third time, I was asked to look after her the first six months or so. "After that I shall go down river until the affair is over," she announced.

"That's nonsense," I objected. "There's no reason why you can't be delivered satisfactorily here."

She stared at me bleakly. "And lose this one as I did the other two because the doctors didn't get here in time? Oh, no! I'm not such a fool as to tempt Fate that way again."

"If your babies had been strong, they might have survived in spite of that misfortune," I told her bluntly. "How do you know that the long journey down river may not be as dangerous to your chances as staying here? In Chungking you'll have your husband present, at least."

She was silent, and I did not press the matter further. A few days later when I stopped in to give her directions for prenatal care, she told me abruptly, "You win, Doctor! I'm going to stay here, provided you swear that nothing will be permitted to keep you away when I send word. If this child dies, it will be the last. I'll never go through this futile suffering and loss again—I've made up my mind to that."

"I'll stick by you if I have to swim the Yangtze," I agreed readily, not dreaming what the promise might cost. "On the other hand, Young Lady, don't you let me catch you breaking a single regulation while you are carrying this child!"

Several times during the months that followed she challenged me with a reminder of that promise. "I've followed your rules faithfully; the rest is up to you!"

I felt perfectly safe in reassuring her. All other deliveries crowding the calendar at that time could, I believed, if emergency arose, be turned over to another Chungking physician. Our own child was not expected until a month after this patient's, and I had no worries on that score.

One afternoon a short time later Maud sent a message to the hospital asking me to stop in at home before making outside calls. When I walked in, she said, "I've been having the queerest feeling for the last hour or so. What do you suppose is the matter?"

Knowing that nothing serious was likely to happen for weeks, I asked, "What did you eat for tiffin?"

"Almost nothing—I wasn't hungry."

On general principles I made an examination, and to my consternation discovered a premature delivery on the way. "Well, since you insist on rushing things," I told her, "it's a good thing I have a fairly free evening."

A few minutes later someone rapped. I opened the door, took a chit from the gateman, and signed the receipt book.

He stood there, adding, "The messenger waits for an answer, *Beh Ih-seng*."

The note announced that my patient in the Hills was having difficulties of her own and begged that I come at once, as had been promised. For the moment I leaned against the door jamb, as breathless from shock as if I had run a race. "Tell the chit-coolie to carry word I'll be there as soon as possible," I ordered and closed the door.

"What's the matter?" asked my wife.

I sat down on the edge of the bed. "Of all the predicaments to be in, this is the worst. Mrs. S—— wants me at once."

There was no need to explain further. Maud knew as well as I did that any trip across the river must be made before dusk—now less than two hours away —and that once there I would have to remain overnight. For a few minutes she lay still with her eyes closed, then looking up, said gamely, "Well, you promised to stick by her and you'd better be starting. Get Lillian and Irene, then see what doctor's in the city to look after me."

The Lillian mentioned was my wife's closest friend in Chungking; the second, while also a friend, had the added advantage of being head nurse at the Canadian Hospital. Our own foreign nurse would have to accompany me on the Hills' case. I dashed off hurried notes to the other Mission doctors, but with no success. Two were up-country and the third on a similar case of his own in the Hills. Strobel refused all obstetrical cases: they were in a field he had never liked and in which he had little skill. Frantically, I ordered chairbearers for the trip to the Hills and decided desperately to resort to the United States gunboat for help. The medical officer there was a personal friend and a capable physician, but for years his experience with women patients had been limited.

I rushed in to bid Maud good-by. She was most uncomfortable. However, even when I told her that "Navy" was our one hope other than a Chinese interne of little experience, she managed to keep her nerve.

"Run along," she ordered. "We're going to have a three-handed bridge game here that will rock the town."

"Send Lao-mi over with a note on the first boat," I told the nurse, and was on my way.

At the river my boatman was directed first to the gunboat. Aboard, I burst in upon the surprised doctor and demanded with forced gaiety, "Want to make a hand at bridge tonight?"

"Yes, I'll be glad to. Things have been fearfully dull out here for the past few days."

"Well, I'll promise you plenty of excitement." Then I explained.

"But, good heavens, man," he exploded, "I haven't handled a delivery in twelve years! I've forgotten the whole technique."

"You'd better do some quick remembering, and what you don't know, ask the nurse."

"But, Basil," he protested, "I just can't . . ."

His words trailed on the air. I was already going down the ladder. "Good luck!" I called back as we pushed off, then muttering to myself, "The Lord have mercy on your soul, if you don't take good care of her!" I slumped into my seat.

Fate was amusing herself at our expense, for my Hills' patient proved to have indigestion, and her baby, a fine healthy boy, was not born for several weeks. Most of the night I strode up and down the veranda outside my room, smoking countless cigarettes and

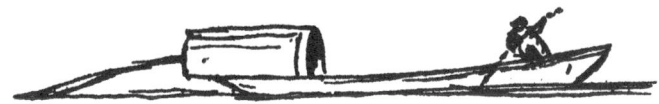

wondering what was happening in that house over at Dai Gia Hang. By daybreak, feeling ten years older than on the previous afternoon, I determined not to wait for Lao-mi's arrival. Time would be saved if I met him on the way, but before I could put this plan into action, the nurse knocked on the door. "Will you come in and have another look, Doctor? The patient seems very miserable."

This proved to be another false alarm, but I was there two hours longer. Lao-mi had not yet appeared, so leaving the nurse in charge, I hurried down to the river bank, only to find him in leisurely discussion with the men on the shore. He came forward slowly to greet me, then passed over the note. I soon learned that a daughter had been born to us around midnight and that mother and child were both doing very well. "Navy," not the Marines, had come to the rescue this time.

"Why didn't you bring this right up to the house?" I demanded. The coolie looked embarrassed. "I knew the child was a girl, *Beh Ih-seng*. Bad enough it was to carry such news; to hurry with it would have been worse."

Grasping his point of view, I said nothing more. Instead, I found an empty space on the next boat. Sitting there in relieved silence and trying to adjust myself to the good news, I overheard one of the crew say to another, "Pity him! His servant just brought word that his firstborn is a girl. Good reason he has to be sad!"

CHAPTER XIV

The Successful Failure

With each passing month in Chungking, I realized more clearly how much the city was enriching my life. This was particularly true with regard to individual contacts. Of these, none was more important than that with Doctor Strobel, whose consuming passion for perfection in his work taught me more than I have any means of estimating.

Exactly one week after our arrival in port an elderly man, stocky and of medium height, with keen blue eyes and sandy hair not yet grayed by age, came into the hospital and asked if I had time to look him over. After introducing himself as Doctor Strobel who had been practicing in Chungking for a good many years, he came at once to the point.

As the examination proceeded, I was momentarily more certain of the man's outstanding ability in medicine. By comparison, my own age and inexperience made the consultation somewhat embarrassing, and I wondered why he had sought out me, the newcomer, for advice. Afterwards I was to learn that long years of professional and social ostracism had kept him from

205

asking favors of other Chungking physicians. It was highly probable that, but for physical wretchedness and perhaps a sudden unconquerable desire for medical discussion, he would not have consulted anyone. While I could tell him nothing about the serious heart condition troubling him, he was enormously interested in discussing the latest therapy in such cases.

At the close of this visit he turned to say hesitatingly, "If you find time to drop in at my home some day, Doctor, you'll be very welcome. I live just around the corner."

After dinner that evening in the Mission group, I asked abruptly, "Why didn't someone tell me there was a physician of Strobel's caliber in Chungking?"

A dead silence settled over the room, then one of the American women found her voice. "How did you happen to meet him, Doctor Basil?"

"He came to my office this morning."

"To your office?" Everybody in the room now stared at me.

"Yes," I answered, completely bewildered by this reaction to a simple question, "is there anything strange about that?"

"Well, in thirty odd years of Chungking residence, this is the third time he has ever entered this compound. The other occasions were a fire and a riot."

"What's the matter—doesn't he like the Methodists?"

"I doubt if he's been even once in most of the other Mission compounds, or for that matter, in many of the business places either," interrupted an older man. "Strobel offers one of those rare instances where community and church out here agree."

"What under heaven is the matter with the man?" I demanded.

A woman who usually said little was the first to answer. "It seems quite possible that there's something the matter with all of us, not just Doctor Strobel, or we'd have used a little more understanding in his case. Personally, I have often wondered how he endures the loneliness of such a life."

"With that big family about him, he can hardly be very lonely," a man broke in impatiently.

"I wasn't referring to the lack of physical companionship. Those who know him say that he has an unusual mind, and his wife and children can hardly satisfy that."

"Oh, nonsense, Miss B——! You're judging him by your own standards. If the man had possessed the right instincts, would he ever have married that coolie woman?"

"Perhaps it was those same right instincts that made him marry her. We all know he didn't have to—certainly a good many foreigners manage to escape responsibility under similar circumstances."

After another remark or two the conversation changed; but these statements, added to my first impression, made me eager to see Doctor Strobel

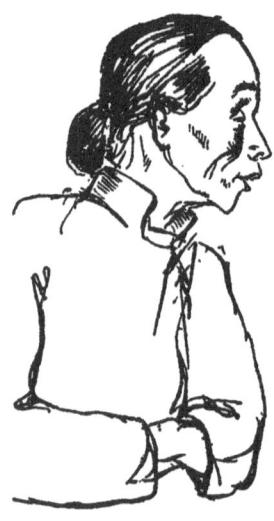

again. Several days later we ran into each other as I was returning from a round of visits on the street, and I seized the moment for calling on him.

It was, I admit frankly, a bit breathtaking to be introduced to the elderly Chinese wife and even more so to meet his children, two golden-haired, blue-eyed Germans and five black-haired, black-eyed Chinese. Once in his office and laboratory, though, this ill-assorted family was swiftly forgotten. Here were to be found all the evidences of a real scientist at work, and I was completely fascinated by what this man had accomplished alone and far from the centers of modern medical achievement.

His primary interest was in blood conditions, and I have never before nor since known anyone able to diagnose so accurately on that basis. Since I was anxious to make the field of intestinal diseases my own, the opportunity to work with a man who knew so much about the blood stream seemed pure luck. Almost daily I dropped in to ask him some question, and he in turn soon acquired the habit of bringing unusual items to me in the hospital.

If the foreign community found it difficult to reconcile this growing intimacy between Strobel and myself with the general attitude, they made no mention of it to me. Even if they had, my own views would have remained unchanged. This outcast was one of medicine's real disciples, and as long as he was willing to teach me,

I had no idea of letting anybody interfere with the arrangement.

As time passed, this professional bond developed into friendship, and one night some impulse made him break off in the middle of an impersonal discussion to tell me about himself. Following graduation in medicine from a German university, he had become an officer in the Prussian Army Medical Corps. Advancement had been rapid—this was easily understood—until factional difficulties caused trouble within the army itself. His own political party lost, and as a result those who belonged to it were demoted in rank. Strobel, young and unmarried, was bitter over this turn of fortune. His pride could not face the sudden disgrace, and the young hothead, in one wild gesture, renounced family, friends, and country to seek a new life at the other end of the world in Mongolia. Eventually drifting down into North China, there he remained until the Boxer Rebellion in 1900. This international difficulty wrecked most of the medical work in that section and, like many other foreigners, he sought refuge in Shanghai.

To his great dismay, far too many of his compatriots had followed the same course. The presence of these other Germans reminded him constantly of all that had been sacrificed in his past. The temptation must have been strong to return to the homeland where family and friends would help him build a new reputation on the ruins of the old. Apparently pride alone stood in the way of this move; yet it was pride that eventually won the fight, and in winning demanded as indemnity a lifetime of exile, grief, and loneliness.

In this second spiritual defeat he closed what he thought was the final door between him and his own kind by heading toward the very heart of China. Beyond those mysterious and almost impassable Gorges of the Upper Yangtze lay Chungking, a city to which few foreigners of any nationality had penetrated and where there was undoubtedly an unlimited field for medical work. Five months after sailing on a houseboat from Shanghai, Doctor Strobel arrived at this chosen destination. Here, alone, and without even a German passport to back him, he daringly planned a career in a section known the length and breadth of the land for its intolerance of strangers. All foreigners were anathema and medical men more than others. Wild rumors that the pink-skinned barbarians from beyond the sea used parts of the human body in making up prescriptions had been circulated all over China, and the more credulous citizens of the West, egged on by their priests and charlatans, considered it a duty to eliminate this menace.

Three times in that first six months of Strobel's residence in Chungking mobs destroyed his office and confiscated most of his few belongings. When, in spite of persecution, he continued to stay on, they put him in a small, unseaworthy boat and set this adrift on the Yangtze's swift current. But Life was not through with their victim. Miraculously enough, the boat washed up on the Little River shore and at night Strobel climbed the heights to the wall, then scaling that, made his way once more into the city.

"Why do you suppose they didn't kill you right off?" I interrupted at this point.

"Perhaps they were afraid to murder a foreigner openly. The success of the International troops over the so-called 'invincible' Boxers in North and Central China had reached even to the West and spread fear. Of course, the Chungkingese could have put an end to *me* without worry, but at that time less familiar with consular routine than they later became, the leaders of the mob did not realize that I was entirely unprotected."

"I can't help wondering why you persisted in tempting Fate here when you might have found a better reception elsewhere."

He smiled a little sadly. "Then it did not seem to matter; also, I was becoming interested in the work here. I had been able to help a few people, and while my enemies seemed to be legion, I knew that these others were my friends. The Chinese have a great gift for friendship, you know," he added, and I remembered that statement vividly, for it was one of the few compliments he ever paid the race voluntarily. Integrity on occasion made him admit that there was much to be admired in this people, but the severe Prussian soldier and scientist was separated from the artistic, easy-going, humor-loving Chinese by so many worlds of thought that a common meeting ground was not easy to find.

By this time in his history, the Chinese must have made up their minds fatalistically to put up with this foreigner whom their repeated attempts had failed to expel. Temporarily let alone, Strobel now set about building up a real practice. The mobs had robbed him of most of his medical equipment, and with amazing ingenuity he improvised substitutes. This inventive ability was characteristic. Compelled to operate unassisted, the man had rigged up contraptions by which he could administer the anesthetic and preside over the field of operation at the same time.

One day on entering his private office unannounced, I found him using a pair of sterile scissors to curet a carbuncle over his own right eye. This was an extremely painful performance, and I demanded, "Why in the world didn't you let me do that for you?"

He countered with a smile, "Don't you find enough work at the hospital?"

Even at that time he had only one medical assistant —a Chungkingese trained in the Chinese technique of pulse taking, which is a highly specialized skill concerned with the whole body. Together they ran efficiently the private hospital of eighteen beds within

Strobel's residence. What commanded admiration was the fact that this man, lacking professional criticism and answerable only to himself, had through the years never sacrificed the principles of good medicine to carelessness or disinterest. This very quality, of course, helped materially in building his reputation. In the beginning, foreign hospitals found it difficult indeed to fill their beds with patients from any but the most desperate and destitute circumstances. The whole of Chinese tradition was against taking a sick person out of his home. From the conservative families, even in my time, it was only the more advanced individual who dared to break with custom by applying at an institution for admittance.

A quarter century earlier, Strobel had accomplished the still greater achievement of persuading Chungkingese to undergo surgical treatment in his private residence. To personal skill there must have been added the most amazing luck, for death under his roof, except in the rarest instances, would certainly have brought the man's West China career to an abrupt end.

Each year a few more foreigners found their way to Chungking and these, in turn, became the German doctor's patients. Hungry for companionship as he was, the same emotional twist that had warped his life previously now made him cold to most friendly overtures. He did, however, have occasional contacts with one or two members of his own race.

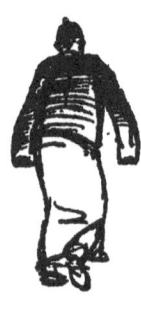

Afterwards one of the older business men in the city told me that while most of the foreigners considered the other a "queer duck," they fully respected his ability and character.

And then Strobel did the one thing calculated to ruin him. Discovering that his Chinese woman servant was going to bear him a child, he married her. To the Europeans this gesture was unforgivably quixotic. For a foreigner separated from the restraining influences of home to indulge in irregularities of conduct was to be expected, they argued tolerantly. But when the offender went the length of legalizing the illicit relationship, he threatened the very foundations of established Western conventions in the East. The Chinese gentry were equally aghast at this mésalliance. For a scholarly scientist to marry a servant was bad enough; for one of their own race, however humble in station, to marry a foreigner was worse.

Warnings to get out now came from both quarters, but again Strobel refused to heed them. There was an abrupt end to the growing friendliness, and while many of the Chinese continued as his patients, Strobel had become the city's most prominent outcast. In his narrative he made little reference to this—it was not the man's nature to ask sympathy—but I had learned enough from other sources and from observation as well to know that few men anywhere have ever lived lonelier lives.

"How you managed to endure your position is beyond me," I told him one night.

He sat staring into the small grate fire before him. "But you understand there was nothing else to do? She had been faithful to my interests from the first." His face clouded with memory. "They used to say to me, 'Strobel, give her a few hundred dollars and pack her off to the country . . . in time the talk will die down.'

"By that time the child was already here and as German in appearance as myself. I would ask them, 'What village will accept her with this foreign infant? Do you know so little of Chinese custom?'"

At this point in his narrative I made no comment. All I could think of was the injustice of bringing into the world those seven racial misfits. In another generation and a different environment it seems quite possible that marriage between Europeans and Orientals may have not only good genetic results, but offer possibilities for happy existence. As yet, this is certainly not true; with all society massed against such unions only misery lies in store for the offspring.

However, it was Strobel the medical man in whom I was most interested. In his laboratory no abstract questions of right or wrong existed; there everything was clear and exact to the most minute detail. His research in blood work was astonishingly complete, for he seemed familiar with every possible change that disease could make in the blood stream.

One morning, Doctor Merton, the English missionary, called me in to look at a case on which he and
another foreign physician in the city could not agree.
Merton thought the patient showed all the symptoms
of typhoid; the other man was equally sure that typhus
was the trouble. While my own findings convinced me
that neither was correct, I had to admit inability to
recognize the real cause.

At once I thought of Strobel. Doctor Merton, who
was not only capable but kind and tolerant beyond
most men, followed the general policy of leaving the
German to himself, and it was not my place as guest
to suggest the other's name. I felt fairly sure, however,
that Strobel, who made the majority of his diagnoses
from blood, would not need to see this patient to find
out what was the matter. I took a blood-smear, and
on my way home carried the slide to him. After careful
study he announced, "An ulcer is at the bottom of
this trouble."

"There was no sign of one."

He shrugged his shoulders and without further ado,
I went back to the patient and got a second, better
smear.

After seeing this, Strobel repeated firmly, "Now I
am sure it is an ulcer. If you cannot find it, then you
have not made a thorough examination."

Nettled by the accusation, I returned once more to
the sick man and this time went over him inch by

inch. At the larynx I decided not to depend on superficial methods, but to use the laryngoscope. With this,
to my great surprise, I found far down at the root of
the tongue an ulcer about the size of a thumbnail.
At once I cauterized. After this treatment had been
repeated four times, the man showed decided improvement and in a few weeks was ready to be discharged.

To Doctor Merton, I admitted frankly where I had
gotten my lead, but I did not mention the case to
Strobel, knowing that he would not bring up the
subject until I did.

On the patient's last day in the hospital, I took
another blood-smear and carried it over to the German.
"This man's been sick but has recovered," was his
immediate verdict. "It looks as if some sort of infection
or ulceration had caused the trouble."

With a sheepish grin I told him the whole story.

Our second summer there, I suffered a sudden
violent intestinal attack. Doctor Strobel was not well
at the time and I hesitated about asking him to make
the hot trip from the city to our Hills cottage. The
three other foreign physicians in port took turns looking
after me. During that first week they injected serum to
the value of two hundred forty dollars (Mexican)—
treatment I myself would have recommended—but in
spite of this I grew steadily worse. In a moment of
lucidity, I insisted on seeing Strobel, and two days
later, returning to full consciousness, I found him at

my bedside. When he would permit talk, I was curious to know what procedure had been followed.

From the night table he lifted a bottle containing a German production that had been used extensively for gangrenous wounds during the World War. Reading in a European medical journal that this was proving effective in certain virulent intestinal disorders, he had used it successfully on several other patients before me. Until then the rest of us in Chungking medical work were unfamiliar with this particular application of the drug; since that time it has become generally accepted and prescribed wherever intestinal diseases are rife.

Near the close of my Chungking experience when Maud, having fought a losing battle with the Szechuen climate, had been forced to return with our small daughter to the States, Strobel made a point of calling on me frequently. One midnight after a brief but silent walk together from the hospital to my residence, he remained to smoke one of his favorite long black cigars. Flicking off an ash, he said without looking up, "I hope you have already given up the idea of a future out here."

Having done nothing of the sort, I asked, "Why do you think that's the only thing for me to do? Six months at home may put Maud in good shape again —what then?"

"Your wife," he went on, carefully weighing each word, "will never be well in this climate. Should she come back, it will be only for short periods at a time. Each separation will be more difficult for both—particularly for you, here where all is alien. Already you miss your family, but the fascination of this work keeps you as yet from facing unpleasant future reality." He paused as if lost in retrospect, then added in a voice rough with emotion, "China's no place for a young foreign man alone—God knows I speak from only the bitterest experience. Go home before the Orient, and this city in particular, eats any more deeply into your life. Two or three years from now it will be too late. Look around you! How many of these foreigners here are willing to stay long at home? You think that stiff-necked pride kept me out here, but I tell you also that the East had already gotten into my blood, as it has in yours. I who ruined my own life ask you not to delay returning to your native land. If you do, you will be a man without a future, with gaze turned always backward toward what has been left."

He never referred to the subject again until I went months later to bid him good-by and to express appreciation for all that he had taught me.

"So you go at last," he remarked gravely. "I shall miss the good medical talks more than ever now, but even so I am glad you are leaving."

"Auf Wiedersehen," I said at parting.

"No, not that," he corrected; "your English 'good-by' is better between us."

I had been home for several years when a former friend from Chungking brought me news of Doctor Strobel's death. His physical condition had grown steadily worse, so I learned, and the man who had drained Life's cup of unhappiness almost to the lees could not find fresh courage with which to face becoming a physical burden. One night, mixing himself a lethal dose, he had gone to bed as usual, and there they found him the next morning.

Characteristically, he had arranged all of his affairs, financial and otherwise, to the last petty detail. His own thrift, together with the Chinese wife's typical racial frugality, had amassed a comfortable sum. There was sufficient to care for her the rest of life and to complete the education of their children. Already the blonde children were in Germany; those distinctively Chinese attended Chungking schools and were planning further training in Shanghai.

In personal association with Doctor Strobel and in the years to follow, my thoughts of him were accompanied always with a sense of irreparable loss to the field of scientific research. Had Fate led him to work in some large medical center, he could have made a much greater contribution to healing than that permitted by his limited life in Chungking. In time, like Osler or Kelly at Johns Hopkins, or the Mayos at Rochester, he also might have been included in the list of Medicine's Immortals.

CHAPTER XV

The Vortex

As time passed, my first revulsion of feeling for Chungking faded completely. I liked filth and bad odors not a whit better than I ever had, but familiarity had now merged these annoyances so successfully into the background that they no longer interfered with my appreciation of the general scene. Perhaps the chief charm of this port for an American lay in the fact that life held no dull moments. Activity was unceasing and ever changing, for in many ways Chungking was a beginning and an end for all China. To the coast, North China, and the entire Yangtze Valley, this city represented the last outpost of trade with Central Asia, while to that vast, mysterious domain beyond that stretched into the heart of the Himalayan ranges the city was the chief gateway to a strange Western world.

Frequently at dusk I would pause on the stretch of city wall behind our compound to look down several hundred feet to the Little River's turmoil of shipping and shore life. Always I had the feeling of standing on the edge of a vortex where West China's life currents were constantly sucked in and spewed out. Towering

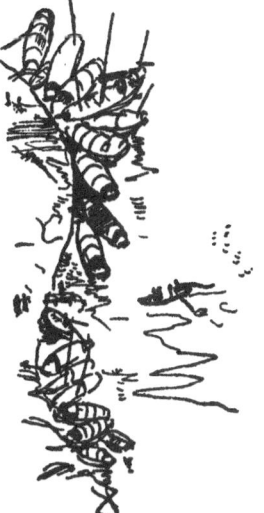

221

over the mass of ramshackle shelters in which so many
of Chungking's poor and outcast managed existence
was the Arsenal, its flickering glare and dull intonations
lending eerie and sinister accent to the whole water
front. A short distance from this was the municipal
slaughterhouse, and the dying squeals of pigs gave the
crowning touch to the inferno-like quality of the
munitions plant.

On the surface of the river floated countless craft
down from inland towns. The boatmen, furling sails or
poling a watery path between wedged traffic, punctuated river chants by hurling good-natured curses at all
in their way. Unheeding, their families went about the
business of normal living aboard, feeding fowls, collecting dried laundry from bamboo poles, or tending the
small charcoal fires under cook-pots.

When I considered the long centuries in which this
scene had remained almost untouched by change, I was
freshly aware of my own country's youth and inexperience. At home in Annapolis we prided ourselves on
age. The town in George Washington's day had been
known as the "Athens of America," antedating Boston's
claim to that title. We had the third oldest college in
the country, and some of the most beautiful of Colonial
architecture, homes in which the founders of the new
nation had met to shape her early policies. We thought
of ourselves as an important part of America's beginnings—all of three hundred years old, a figure which

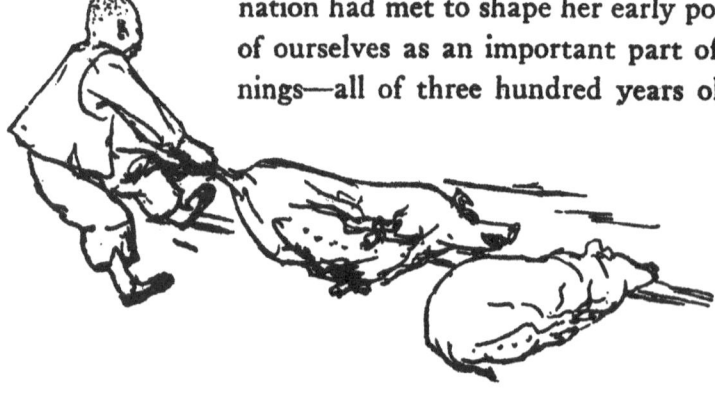

suddenly became absurd when I recalled the traditional founding of Chungking in 2200 B.C.

On a number of occasions I tried to authenticate this figure, which lay in the so-called mythical era of Chinese history. Scholars of the old school readily accepted this early date; but the modern students, debunking every year of which there was not archeological proof, believed the end of the Later Han Dynasty about A.D. 200 more nearly correct.

A good deal of my information came from a returned student who frequented the tea-house nearest the hospital. After taking honors in law at a great American university, he had gone home to Chungking for the purpose of establishing a practice along Western lines. As might have been expected, he had met defeat in every court, and when I knew him, the man in his early thirties had become a ne'er-do-well about town, finding his only solace in opium. To me he presented an outstanding example of foolishly wasted material. A number of other professions would have offered opportunity for personal success and civic service, but to tackle Chinese law single-handed in the interior seemed as futile as Don Quixote's tilting at windmills. Watching him there at the tea-house table, with his attention turned inward on frustrated ambition and his original dapper grooming becoming daily more slovenly, I was reminded of the hundreds of other Chinese returned students like him. Many of these as a result of unwise training and an overemphasis on Westernization, find themselves suspended between two civilizations and are unable to plant their feet firmly on either.

My visits to the tea-house were almost always limited in time, but whenever I found this patron free of opium, I would sit down at his table, give my order, and then urge him to expression. Often these foreign-educated youths sacrifice knowledge of their own history and learning in the pursuit of Occidental studies. This was not true in his case, and he sketched in bit by bit a fairly comprehensive outline of China's past and present. The discovery of the "Oracle bones" in North China and the archeological rumors that these were establishing, beyond a shadow of a doubt, the existence of the Shang Dynasty fifteen hundred or more years before Christ interested him greatly.

However, like most Szechuenese, his knowledge about his native locale was hazy. Szechuen, I had heard, was a mixture of Chinese from other sections with possibly a strain from aboriginal tribes. Racial pride made him discount the theory of tribal relationships, though he was quite willing to agree that early settlers were predominantly Shantung people who had migrated West during a severe period of drought. This, it was argued, accounted for the similarities in the Szechuen and North China dialects. (The official Mandarin is spoken all over North, Central, and West

China, but it is subjected to numerous minor changes in each of the three sections.) Regarding Chungking itself, he knew little more than the others I had questioned.

"Do you think it true that the city wall has been rebuilt four or five times?" I asked.

"Yes, but not in entirety."

"Even though the place is strategically and firmly located," I continued, "it seems strange that the small area of the site did not deter those early builders."

"They soon found ways to overcome that—look at Kiang-beh! And what other city in this land builds stories on top of each other?"

"What led to Kiang-beh? Certainly no Chungkingese would live outside the city wall if he could afford not to do so."

"That's the answer, Doctor. Excessive taxation within the city forced a great many citizens in moderate circumstances to find living quarters elsewhere. These crossed to Kiang-beh and there, as the new community enlarged, built a wall of their own."

Once or twice I turned the subject from impersonal topics to himself. "Since modern legal practice in Chungking is not feasible, why don't you teach English in a Government School?"

"You forget, *Beh Ih-seng*, that all of my difficulties have been with officials, and they control such posts."

His sudden sharp glance was a warning, but knowing that the real answer still lay hidden, I dared to prod.

"Some of the officials are my friends. If you'd like me to speak to them . . ."

"I am most unworthy of your great interest," he replied automatically, then emotion swept away courteous restraint. "Am I then, with my degrees and honors, to accept a position that any freshman from Chengtu (the provincial capital where the university was located) might fill? My 'face' would be gone forever."

"Oh, that's foolish! You've had enough foreign training to know that some things are more important than 'face.' "

With dignity he put an end to my meddling. "Foreign training, yes; but the fact remains, *Beh Ih-seng*, that I am a Chinese."

After a time I missed him from his usual place, and what eventually became of him I never learned.

When I talked with Strobel about Chungking, he had said thoughtfully, "A strange city, drawing men like a gold mine. Though it's this great West and not the city from which the wealth is extracted. Chungking by taxes and customs duties merely seizes for her own a bit of the choicest ore from every bag passing through her gates."

"So, you, too, admit the place has personality," I commented drily. "I thought such flights of fancy characteristic only of young Americans who are particularly susceptible to the charms of what is alien and old."

"The attraction of the alien perhaps—but what has age to do with it? I have known Europe's ancient spots and Peking. Once in that old capital, you will understand that age is not the answer to this riddle. Peking has beauty. When you have seen her lacquered roofs and marble palaces, the broad roads, and bright blue sky, you will recall this city's filth and ugliness. A little ashamed you will say, 'I must have been out of my mind to see anything in Chungking!' "

"Too many foreigners live there," I objected.

"Not so fast! You have not yet seen Peking. When you do, you may find yourself playing with the idea of settling down in that invigorating climate. The Rockefeller Hospital, from all reports, is magnificently equipped for research," he threw out as a lure.

"Then what?"

"Then you take the train to Hankow and board the first Upper River steamer for Chungking."

"You might at least furnish the reason."

He shook his gray head. "Neither I, nor any other foreigner who chooses to remain in this *Höllenloch* (hellhole), can tell you that."

When I tried to analyze the facts, there seemed no valid reason for foreigners to waste any depth of feeling on Chungking. During the years their group had fluctuated between twenty and two hundred members, an infinitesimal fraction of the city's population. Each one of the outsiders in time acquired a number of Chinese friends and acquaintances, but to the great mass of citizens he remained an undesirable, a "foreign dog," who would always bear watching. The city made no attempt to conceal this suspicious attitude, and Westerners met it in innumerable subtle annoyances. When these did not wear him out, the climate usually stepped in and finished the job.

On the other hand, there was no apparent reason for the Chungkingese to like the foreigners. Few of them believed that the Mission institutions had no ulterior motives behind their altruistic programs; too many pages of modern Chinese history gave the lie to this idea. In most instances the foreigner's religion had merely opened the way to trade, and between trade and gunboats the step had been a short one.

Superficially we were unlike them in every way— physical appearance, dress, speech, and customs. The swift resentment I felt when Chinese street urchins yelled "*Yang Kuei tz!*" (Foreign devil), after me or spat on my shadow illustrated man's inconsistency. Not so many years earlier, my companions and I had stuck our heads in the doorway of the Annapolis Chinese laundry and had taunted, "Chink-chink-China-man eat dead rats!" This had been the least of inflicted torments; yet that solitary figure had stuck industriously at his job enduring slights and destructive pranks with the bleak certainty that when we were gone, he would have to face the same persecution from

other boys who were already growing up to fill our
places.

The chief difference between the foreigners in China
and those scattered Orientals in America was that we
made demands and they did not. The same arrogant
twist that makes the white race, wherever it goes, feel
that it exists under a special dispensation was not
absent from the Chungking scene. That foreigner was
rare who was not conscious of the Stars and Stripes,
the Union Jack, or the Tricolor waving protectingly
about him when he asked for some special privilege
that the native Chinese could not hope to claim.

When difficulties arose, Occidentals, whatever their
national differences normally, at once became blood-
brothers. This was only partially explained by the fact
that trouble for one foreigner often meant trouble for
all of them. Chungking had, it was true, staged a
number of anti-foreign riots in her time. The worst of
these was in 1886 when most of the foreign property
was destroyed. The port was not opened to Western
trade until 1891, and this traffic was limited to junk
and houseboat. Only in 1898 did the first small steamer
fight its hazardous way through the Gorges from
Ichang and make the city more accessible to Americans
and Europeans.

The resulting contacts did much to break down
barriers between Chungkingese and foreigners, but even
so, I had the feeling that the two remained constantly
16

on guard like wary fencers ready to parry every possible thrust. Nevertheless, each side managed to "slip one over" occasionally on the other.

General Den, the Chungking warlord, wishing to advertise his familiarity with modern technical methods of warfare, invited officials and militarists from all over the province to view a bombing demonstration on a field outside Chungking. For this purpose he had bought an antiquated crate, had it shipped up river, and reassembled locally. Then hiring a German aviator from Shanghai to fly it, he appointed a young, insufficiently trained Chinese as co-pilot.

At the specified hour, Den, his guests, and a mob of Chungkingese met at the field for the performance. The section over which the plane was to circle had been carefully marked off, and in the center was located the spot where the bomb was supposed to fall.

Once up in the air, the German found his entire attention and effort would be needed to keep the wreck flying, and the pilot would have to look after the bombs without advice from him. Made responsible for gauging the machine's speed and position with relation to the field, the young Chinese nervously miscalculated and catapulted the first bomb into the midst of the crowd.

The result was horrible beyond description. Victims were rushed into the hospital, but approximately ninety per cent of these were beyond help. When the plane landed, both men were seized and taken to the *Yamen*. At once a dozen different rumors were circulated explaining the accident, but the one given above seemed the most plausible to me.

Chungking public opinion ran high. A number of her citizens had been killed in the tragedy, and the populace demanded immediate death penalties for both individuals involved. The young Chinese was doomed, of course, and there was little reason to think that the German would not have to share the other's fate. Parnell, who had previously known the aviator in Shanghai, came in to dinner that night with a long face; he felt that there was little hope of the German's saving his skin.

At the time the German consul's wife was in an unpromising pregnant condition, and I had been paying daily visits to their home. When I reached there the next morning, I noticed at once the air of secrecy and strain about the household and supposed this due to worry over their compatriot's trouble, as it turned out to be. With the professional call concluded, I started down the hall to the stairs and, to my astonishment, was halted at the top of the flight by no other than Parnell.

"What are you doing over here in business hours?" I exclaimed.

Without a word he led me into another room down the corridor and closed the door firmly behind us. Inside sat the Consul, a half dozen of the business men in Chungking's German community, and a stranger, who was at once introduced to me as the aviator. His unexpected presence was explained promptly for my benefit. The Consul and the officials at the *Yamen* had spent most of the previous night, so I learned, arguing what was to be done with the prisoner. It may be that the *Yamen*, fully aware of the international dangers connected with holding this foreigner, decided finally that it might be best to turn the job over to the German Consul. Then if the Chungkingese chose to take the aviator from his own government's representative, the Chinese officials could not be held to account for another foreign incident.

But whatever the reason, the transfer had been made. Dressed in Chinese robes, the flyer had been smuggled in a closed chair from one official residence to the other through streets still thronged by angry citizens. Listening to this, I could find no great advantage in the move. In time his escape from the *Yamen* was bound to leak out, and the mob would turn at once to the German residences for their quarry. It would be much easier to force entrance to one of these buildings than to the *Yamen*, and I said so.

"But that's where you come in, George," Parnell replied. "We've been discussing how to get O—— out of town without delay, and I told them you were just the one to help us."

"I? What do you mean?"

"There's a steamer sailing at dawn," he hurried on. "If he can reach that second landing on the Yangtze in time, the ship will pick him up. But the problem is to get him down there; for that we've got to have a boat. The German launch is undergoing engine repairs and the only other one available is the Oil Company's. You see!"

"No, I don't," was my retort.

"Well it's plain enough, Heaven knows. All you do is write a chit to your friend, the manager, and he'll lend you his boat."

"He's gone upcountry for a week, and I don't believe he'd lend it for this purpose, if he were here."

"All the better then! His Chinese compradore would not think of refusing you."

"You mean I'm to ask him to do what I feel sure his boss wouldn't like? Look, Dave, I'm as sorry as anybody else for your friend's predicament, but it's a problem for the German and Chinese governments to settle between them. That Oil Company launch flies the American flag, and if caught, would certainly be in a nice mess with the authorities." So far this conversation, while limited to the two of us, had been loud enough for all present to hear. Now I added in an undertone, "If the Consul got this fellow out on bond, how does he dare to risk letting him get away?"

"Let him worry about that! There must have been some sort of understanding between him and the officials. Do you think they didn't realize that this would follow?"

"Well, why do you have to have a motorboat? Why not use a sampan?"

"Too much danger of recognition from the local boatmen."

"If he arrived the day of the flight and made his one public appearance at the field in flying uniform, helmet, and goggles, how many Chungkingese ever really saw him?"

The refugee now spoke up. "That's what I suggested before you came in, Doctor. If we can wait until night, I might be able to make it in an ordinary business suit."

"But boatmen won't travel at night—it's too dangerous," objected one of his countrymen.

Chungking had at this time been enjoying several unusually clear days and moonlit nights. "If the mists do not rise this evening, I know boatmen who'll take you." I mentioned the men who, for a good price, sometimes ferried me to Kiang-beh for night emergency calls. "You and Parnell can meet me outside our compound," I went on, "at nine o'clock and we'll go down to the shore together. The boatman will know only that you are my guest who has important business at the landing. I don't believe there will be any difficulties."

This arrangement was seized upon, and I left almost at once, wondering a little too late if I had voluntarily created special trouble for myself. My chief question

had to do with the Chinese government. It seemed
doubtful that they had not counted the possible cost
of letting this prisoner escape. Chinese citizenry were
proverbially long-suffering, but every once in a while
the straw was added that broke the camel's back.
When that happened, officials were as likely to suffer
at the hands of the infuriated people as was anybody
else. However, the authorities were probably much
better able to gauge the temperature of public feeling
in this instance than I, and, as Parnell had suggested,
they and the German Consul were the ones to do the
worrying. I could imagine that the aviator was spending his time praying for the anticipated moonlight.

This eventually arrived. At the appointed hour and
place the three of us met and went down to the shore
where we had to wait for about ten minutes before the
boatman came. Chungking and its environs had already
taken to bed. From the innumerable small craft
anchored offshore came the occasional sound of lowered
voices, but the noisy activities of the day were at an
end. It was very peaceful there in the moonlight as we
stood listening to the rise and fall of the hundreds of
small hulls that lay on the Lin's bosom. Then suddenly
a sharp, unearthly glare lit up the opposite bank and
from above our heads rattled the unexpected fire from
a machine gun.

For a second Parnell and I, entirely familiar with
such sights and sounds, were nonetheless startled; the

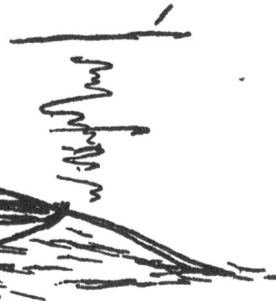

escaping flyer must surely have thought that doom had overtaken him. We explained at once. On the Kiang-beh mud flats the Chungking arsenal had set up a large target for machine-gun practice from our side of the river. To light up this bull's-eye on dark nights, they occasionally sent up rocket flares. A good many of the arsenal's activities seemed without rime or reason, but why they had chosen to waste a rocket in bright moonlight was hard to fathom. Certainly it was not concern for the safety of Kiang-beh citizens, for these were only too frequently the casualties resulting from poor aim.

The sampan finally arrived. Placing the passenger aboard, we wished him "Good luck!" and watched the craft make its way into midstream. Next morning the steamer picked up the refugee as previously arranged and carried him down river. While a wave of excited talk swept the city following the discovery of his escape, no punitive action ensued on the part of people or officials. I was nevertheless glad that my own name was not once linked with the affair, though at times I could not help but wonder if those Lin River boatmen connected their special passenger with the figure of the missing aviator. If they did, no one was ever likely to know. They had their own reasons for keeping silent, and personally I could think of a great many more discreet subjects for any future conversations I might have with them.

CHAPTER XVI

Attempts to Scale the Dragon

At the beginning of my third year in Chungking, General Den, the *Tuchun* (Military Governor) sent a note inviting me to see him professionally in his home. Having learned much earlier to adapt modern medical procedure to the needs of Chinese officials, I had no hesitation about making this call. On arrival, however, I found the General already in the hands of two old-fashioned Chinese doctors. The professional problem did not bother the sick man at all; used to running things his own way, he now asked me hoarsely to give the others suggestions. For the first few minutes the situation seemed charged with dynamite, but after an hour had been wasted in much ceremonial palaver, the two physicians assured me that I would confer a great favor on them by examining the patient in the foreign manner.

General Den was lying on a cane bed, over a large chest filled with ice—an arrangement similar to the North China *kang* (oven bed), in which a banked fire keeps the sleeper warm. I found acute kidney complications, as in so many well-to-do Chinese, but what bothered me most was a badly congested chest. In spite of high temperature, his feet and hands were blue with cold, and it seemed likely that if he continued on ice, a bronchial pneumonia might soon develop.

The other doctors knew quite as well as I that the kidneys were affected, so I asked them politely, "Is it Chinese custom to use ice for this disease?"

"No. In this case we wish to lessen the body's heat."

This wasn't so far off the track for normal reduction of temperature, but they did not seem to realize that with the accompanying bronchial infection the temperature would keep right on going up. I explained as diplomatically as possible that the foreign method would be to keep this patient dry and warm; also, that instead of forcing food and restricting liquids as they had been doing, I would reverse the process. These changes in treatment were entirely agreeable to them, they informed me, and thereby gracefully shifted full responsibility to my shoulders for the patient's future condition.

"This patient takes opium, doesn't he?" I asked in the course of questioning.

"Oh, no, *Beh Ih-seng*, His Excellency does not have so evil a habit!" they protested in shocked voices.

To save their "faces," I replied, "You must have misunderstood me. When I noticed physical signs of the drug, it was not my meaning to say that General Den uses it in that fashion, but perhaps as a medicine."

Without blinking an eyelash, they admitted gravely, "It is true, we misunderstood, Honorable Doctor. His Excellency has bowel trouble, and we advised him to smoke a little for relief."

When opium was used for medication, the custom was to give it by mouth; smoking was the form in which addicts took it. Sensing that I might know this also, they hastened to add, "His Excellency does not like to swallow the drug, therefore he smokes it."

"When the patient's intestinal trouble requires the drug, it is, of course, all right to let him have a little," I assured them. Supported in this statement by good medical theory, I then let the matter drop.

But the Chinese did not. At the end of this visit, servants brought in a new and complete set of opium smoking equipment and offered it to me instead of the customary bowl of tea. Since I had raised so little objection to General Den's use of it, they undoubtedly thought I enjoyed a pipeful of my own on occasion.

A short time after the General's recovery, his military aide in charge of education called on me one afternoon.

"*Beh Ih-seng*, General Den sent me here," he announced after the usual preliminaries. "He wishes me to ask a great favor. If you will teach the students in the schools how to become strong men, His Excellency will be glad to pay well for your services."

This came as a great surprise. The General, a crafty old warlord, was not noted for his interest in public welfare, and I wondered about his motive. Also, lecturing to all the students in the Government high schools seemed a large order in an already crowded schedule. On the other hand, some form of Public Health work was needed in Chungking above all things, and this offer seemed to be an opening wedge. I accepted and told him to inform General Den that the hospital would be glad to co-operate without charge in such a good cause.

In Chungking proper there was no hall sufficiently large to hold these groups of several hundred each, so I went over to Kiang-Beh (North of the River) three times a week. This town was an overflow community from the greater city, and its newer Government School had a large assembly room..From the first the students seemed interested and were always ready to engage in discussion. No matter what the subject was, someone would jump up to quote from Chinese tradition concerning it.

That regular hours, bathing, tooth brushing, and exercising all had their places in Confucian ritual, I soon learned. "After the rooster crows the third time, no man should lie in bed," they would quote. "On rising, a man must wash face and teeth. By moving his bed about the room he can exercise his body. When this has been done, he should step outside and there breathe the fresh air deeply many times." These health rules, incorporated from material on Right

Living centuries old were not a bad foundation on which to develop modern hygiene. It was in the field of preventive medicine that Chinese and Western theories really clashed.

With the assistance of colorful charts and pamphlets, I explained the importance of keeping hands clean; of protecting food from dust; and of using care in expectorating, and in the handling of body disposals. "Most necessary is it to keep your breathing passage open and free of dust," I added. "You have by nature a number of small hairs within the nose. These sift foreign elements at entrance and prevent their advance into more delicate channels. When the nose is stopped up, you cannot breathe well and that is bad for the whole body."

"What you say, *Beh-Ih-seng*, may be true of Americans," someone contradicted, "but not of Chinese. The chief use of our noses is to smell. When they are stopped up, we breathe through the mouth."

Pigeonholing this for further explanation at some later date, I would find myself in equal difficulty elsewhere.

"You say, 'by nature' we have hairs in nose, *Beh Ih-seng;* nature is what meaning?"

Usually I spoke in my own limited Chinese, but a foreigner with language background was present most of the time to help out in awkward moments. This was one of them.

"Nature means those qualities of mind and body with which man comes into the world," I would have the interpreter tell them. "Physically, it is his ability to grow, to increase strength, to resist and fight disease, or the opposite of all these. We say it is man's nature to breathe through lungs and nasal passages; it is a fish's nature to breathe through gills. Mentally, man's nature is the way he thinks and acts when he is not restrained by rules. It is one man's nature to be good and kind, we say; it is another's to be bad and cruel. Now do you understand."

"Yes, yes, *Beh Ih-seng!* Nature means *feng-shui.*"

Feng-shui—elemental spirits of good and evil and their effect on life, I would translate slowly for myself. This was close, but not close enough. In desperation I would turn to my standby, "M——, for Heaven's sake you tell them what nature means!"

"I'll be hanged if I know how to explain it!" Scratching his head, he would try to clarify my earlier attempt.

While the two foreigners harangued over this common English expression, the assembly remained politely quiet. After a session or two, I learned to avoid such abstract terms as I would the plague.

"The West China people have received great nutritional gifts in rice and oranges," I would continue along another line, "and the warm, moist climate makes green vegetables grow in profusion. This Szechuen plain of yours has been known to yield seven crops a year. Where the land is so rich as this, there is no need to use human excrement for fertilization!"

"But, *Beh Ih-seng,* if farmers did not use night-soil, land would not be so rich and fields would not give so many crops," they would chorus in protest.

"Using night-soil for food growing is what gives most of you dysentery. Would it not be better to have fewer, but cleaner crops?"

"Whether from dysentery or hunger, some men must die, Doctor. *Muh iu fa tz!*"

In the hope of breaking down such attitudes, a fresh attack would be tried. "Soon you will marry. If your wife bears a son, everyone under your roof will be happy. The mother, grandmother, wet-nurse, you, yourself—all will handle the baby constantly. If his small hand grips your fingers and finds them unclean, that dirt will be transferred into his mouth. Perhaps your 'slops' coolie has buckets that drip; the flies that find these drops of filth on the floor may travel next to your son's face. Because the baby grabs playfully at a long, green cucumber, your wife lets him have it to chew on. Then, some day when the child is perhaps two years old (One year by Western count; Chinese reckoning credits a child with a year of life at birth) he becomes ill with dysentery and, to your whole family's intense sorrow, dies. Soiled hands, flies, the raw cucumber from a field fertilized by night-soil, any one of these may have caused his death. All of them with a little care could have been avoided."

When lessons were brought home to them in this fashion, the students listened with grave attention. For the moment they were young crusaders in the fight against filth and disease. A few moments later, crossing the curb between lecture hall and street, they would find themselves once more in a scoffing and unbelieving world, where custom and tradition were stoutly allied against all that was foreign and new. Even in the face of such opposition though, their leaven of interest worked. Adults began to attend the lectures; teachers, professional men, and army officers now occupied many of the benches. Following the talk, the meetings became open forums, for the Chinese love argument and are particularly good at rebuttal.

"You say, Doctor, that in America there are laws against spitting, polluted water, open sewage, and many other things that spread disease. Since that is true, Americans should be stronger than Chinese and live to greater age, not so?"

This was a poser, for all Chinese, I believe, barring the presence of infections and elemental calamities, might live naturally to be a hundred. Almost everything about their way of life is conducive to longevity. Their working days are much longer than ours, but no energy is wasted trying to live at the unnatural tempo of most Westerners. They work steadily though without hurry.

When they relax, they do so completely. If a task should remain unfinished tonight, *muh iu fa tz!* The workman has done the best he could for this day—can more be expected? He will finish it tomorrow. Neither threat nor bribe will make him slight the job. As an apprentice he learned to be painstaking and thorough. Now that he is a journeyman, is there any reason why he should forget all his training and become careless, simply because a mad foreigner wishes the work finished before it is possible? What matters one day or another, so that the task is done well?

Everything in Chinese life follows the same pattern. When a man eats, he does it slowly and with enjoyment. In a land where the population is enormous and famine in some sections frequent, food is a precious commodity and should be appreciated in the eating. One of their proverbs says, "If you must hurry a servant, do so at his work, not at his meal."

The average Chinese knows how to manipulate his body to the best advantage. Coolies carry terrific loads for long distances, but these are so adjusted that the minimum of muscular strain is required.

When he is ready to sleep, neither the presence of noise nor activity interferes with that purpose. His nervous system is a servant to obey commands; in most Westerners it is a tyrant that must be pampered to be endured. High blood pressure, heart disease, even appendix and gall bladder troubles—all of which take

17

a terrific toll in American life—are almost never seen among Chinese. In my personal experience, necessity for surgical intervention in China and in America seemed proportionately about one to a hundred.

Accordingly, when questioned in the lecture room concerning relative life span in the two peoples, I would compromise. "Chinese probably live longer than Americans, for the centuries have taught you to live more sanely. We are a young nation and with customary youthful greed snatch at living. This sacrifice of energy shortens life for many of us. On the other hand, more of our babies live to become adults."

This point would be discussed at length—some requesting concrete formulas for improving conditions; others taking the defeatist attitude, so typical of Old China, that life had gone on this way throughout history, and if good could have been accomplished by changing, their ancestors would certainly have done so.

"If one of your communities might be made, over a period of even a few years, to observe the simple rules of cleanliness and sanitation, you would be astonished by the results. More Szechuenese suffer from tuberculosis and dysentery than from anything else. These are two diseases that modern science knows how to control."

"Some Americans, *Beh Ih-seng*, have these diseases, is it not so? Why is that?"

"Yes, but they are not permitted to spread them at will among members of their families and friends. Some day it is hoped they will be as rare as smallpox in our country."

"Smallpox, *puh iao ching* (Unimportant)!" they would interrupt with a shrug. Almost every Chinese has smallpox at some time in life, but having built up a degree of racial immunity, none of them fear the "Heavenly Flower," a picturesque term for the disease that the foreigner finds difficult to appreciate. On the other hand, measles, supposed to have been carried to China by foreigners, terrifies them and with good reason, for it usually results in death.

At the end of this lecture course, I invited the adults to visit the hospital's tubercular clinic where they might see for themselves modern methods of treatment. Many of them accepted, and through the following months these interested observers were given opportunity to note the beneficial effect of rest, good food, fresh air, cod-liver oil, and orange juice on a victim of this disease.

Leaving our corridors, they went out to spread the gospel of modern medicine through Chungking's highways and byways. In 1938, when Generalissimo Chiang Kai-shek made the city his headquarters, one of his first moves was to promote a strenuous program of Public Health. I like to think that the young Chinese physicians, alert and foreign trained, who conducted this, found some fruit from seeds that had been sown years earlier.

One question that troubled me particularly was why amoebic dysentery seemed more virulent in the countryside than in the city. Hospital duty did not permit me to go far afield, but whenever possible, I slipped off to rural villages to study living conditions for the sake of contrasting them with urban ones. In both types of community the contributing, major factors to this disease were the same familiar trio: human ordure for fertilization; flies; and careless handling of food.

I soon discovered that the Chungkingese had a great advantage over the country people where direct exposure was concerned. Every tiny farm had its *kong*, a large pottery vat from three to four feet high in which to store night-soil generously diluted by water. When fertilization was needed for the ground, the farmer filled two buckets from the *kong* and carried them on a shoulder pole to the fields. There with the aid of a large wooden dipper, the semi-solid mass was deposited around each young plant. If he and his family miraculously escaped contamination from soiled hands and garments, the flies finished the job.

Protected from these evils, the city dweller still had to face two possibilities of infection: first, by the polluted vegetables the countryman had sold him; second, from uncleanliness in the preparation and serving. The custom of eating food steaming hot is their greatest protective agent. It is, unfortunately, their only one.

The Chungkingese were much more likely to seek medical advice soon after the symptoms of an attack became manifest; the farmer was usually his own doctor. Accustomed to weariness and discomfort, he often reached the point of exhaustion before eating a little opium, the time-honored specific not only in the Orient but in the Occident for diarrhea. This drug, smothering the organism temporarily, did nothing toward destroying it. The patient went on working and dosing; then one day the infection reached his liver and, developing an abscess, killed him.

To find so many liver abscesses was a rare privilege for the physician, although hard on the sufferers. Those cases of amoebic dysentery that are brought to the doctor's attention in America seldom have the liver complication. While no permanent cure has yet been found for this disease, proper medication at regular intervals and a built-up resistance checks its advance.

At first I tried a major operation on such cases, but with little success. After these discouraging attempts, I settled down to the much simpler process of draining the superficial abscess through the lateral wall. This resulted in a number of recoveries.

For the usual amoebic dysentery attack I found the generally accepted drug, emetine, a poor stick on which to lean. This form of ipecac, while it did check the complaint to some extent, was usually very hard on the sufferer, adding nausea, sick headache, and other unpleasant reactions of its own. Furthermore, its effect lasted too short a time. I began to use yatren, or its associated compounds under other trade names more and more frequently, giving it orally fifteen grains every four hours, and on alternate days, administering a rectal solution of thirty grains in water, to be retained from six to ten hours. The only really unpleasant reaction of the drug after successive doses was to excite the nervous system.

Aside from this, the patient almost invariably admitted feeling stronger and clearer headed after the first day of treatment. I have heard physicians object to the use of yatren on the ground that for the first two or three days the active dysentery seems to increase rather than decrease. This is usually true enough but after that healing begins, and unless the patient's resistance is extremely low, he can go for a period of six months without further treatment. In my opinion it is inadvisable to make this resting period longer.

In connection with any therapy for this disease, I cannot stress too greatly the use of ice. Its effect is amazingly prompt in slowing the motility of the intestines and in preventing the spread of ulcers as well. It seems to afford the patient almost indescribable relief, and the Chungkingese, ordinarily averse to touching ice, a scarce article in West China, was only too glad to use over an ulceration his share from the hospital's electric refrigeration plant.

On a country trip when I had to remain overnight, I had the worst of all my experiences with Chinese inns. We were a good distance away from Chungking; a cold drizzling rain had set in, and the chair-bearers preferred to wait until daylight before starting homeward. In such hostelries, it is nothing unusual to find the *mao-fang* (open toilet) and pigpen separated from one's sleeping quarters by only the thinnest partition, but in this instance they occupied one end of the guest room itself.

As had been predicted on my first visit to the hospital, I had gradually grown accustomed to unpleasant odors. In this place, however, smells seemed to have reached a "new high." Moreover, the establishment was evidently licensed to dispense opium, for the bunks to accommodate the users of the drug were built all along one wall. While Lao-mi set up my cot in an empty one of these and adjusted the mosquito net, I began to study some of the other travelers. In the bunk next mine was a man with the dead white, hairless skin that denoted leprosy, even without the additional testimony his sharp-pointed fingers supplied.

Spasms of coughing across the aisle made me glance in that direction. There, looking as much like a living corpse as anything I have ever seen, was a victim of pulmonary tuberculosis. He must have been eighty years old, and I wondered how his body, smaller than a child's, could possibly have held him up under the strain of journeying anywhere, however short the distance. Each time he spat on the floor it seemed likely to be his last act.

Somewhat discouraged by the surroundings, I did not attempt to remove garments. With the building closed against the night, no fresh air entered to relieve the fetid mixture we were breathing, and beneath the net it was stifling. After a time, I threw this aside and eventually dozed off into sleep broken by the monotonous sound of snores and groans.

A sharp, stabbing pain in the ear woke me in time to see the great rat that had bitten me leap nimbly across the room. Wiping blood from my cheek, I tucked the net once more around me but after an hour or so, again discarded it, deciding that the risk of rat bite was no worse than that of suffocating.

When the usual four o'clock call roused me, my whole body burned and stung. Muscles were stiff and taut, and painfully I began the undressing that had not been done before retiring. Several peculiar streaks of red stretched over my body. These were easily recognized as centipede stings. Every once in a while some patient came to the hospital suffering from these venomous bites, which in effect resembled formic acid burns and may have been just that. I washed my own at once in ammonia water, but for a number of days the secondary infection they produced continued to poison my system.

One peculiarity I had noticed in connection with such stings in others: those administered on the back caused the most severe pain by directly affecting the kidneys; and one patient died in the hospital as a result. Due to hot weather he had slept practically naked, and the centipede, crawling all over him, had stung again and again.

Chinese fear these creatures much more than they do spiders or snakes. At first, the newcomer smiles over this native fear, thinking it rather foolish; in time, from sad, personal experience, he learns to understand.

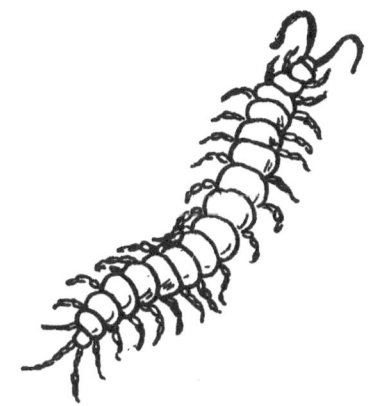

CHAPTER XVII

Starring Without Rehearsal

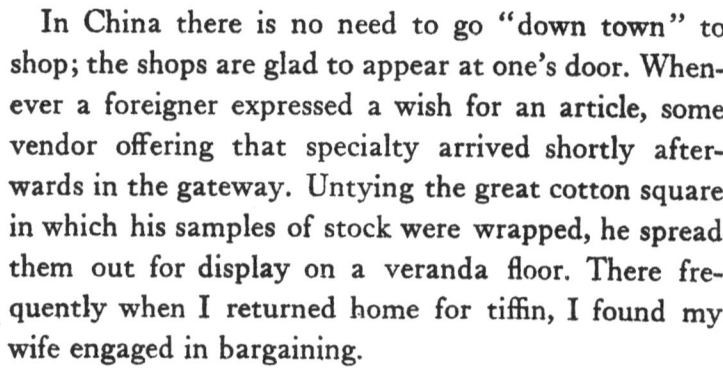

In China there is no need to go "down town" to shop; the shops are glad to appear at one's door. Whenever a foreigner expressed a wish for an article, some vendor offering that specialty arrived shortly afterwards in the gateway. Untying the great cotton square in which his samples of stock were wrapped, he spread them out for display on a veranda floor. There frequently when I returned home for tiffin, I found my wife engaged in bargaining.

Such affairs are never of short duration, for the Chinese take the greatest delight in matching wits financially. In this instance where the buyer had only a few words of the language and the vendor practically no English, transactions took longer than ordinary. We had both acquired the native habit of pretending not to be interested in the thing we really wanted. If Maud seemed to be concentrating on a pair of candlesticks, I asked under my breath, "What is it you wish —that incense burner?"

"Mnh!" she assented, without even the flicker of an eyelash toward the object, while the vendor, thoroughly familiar with such tactics, had a silent guessing game of his own.

Like most foreign men, after having looked over the stock and listened to the argument for several minutes, I found my attention wandering. "Is tiffin ready?"

Hustled thus abruptly from high finance to domesticity, my wife would look up with a puzzled frown. "How do I tell him that incense burner is poorly cut?"

When this speech had been worked out, presented in challenge, and politely refuted, Maud again simulated interest in the candlesticks.

"I'll bet this fellow has liver trouble," I ventured appraisingly. "Look at his saffron skin and discolored eye whites!" My wife turned a deaf ear, so my next sentence was directed where it would count. "Brass-seller, does your stomach ache?"

Startled by so unexpected an attack, the man stammered, "No—yes—how did you know, *Beh Ih-seng?*"

"Your head goes round and round, not so?"

"Truly!"

"What medicine do you eat?"

"Ox-gall in rice wine."

"Does it make you better?"

He hesitated. "Sometimes."

"Not always?"

"No-o!"

"Then why take it?"

"It's cheaper than bear's gall or elephant hide."

These oddities were commonly used for liver congestion in China, as were pig's liver, bamboo buds, and herbs. In research work at Peking and Shanghai, it was being discovered that boiled donkey hide, used extensively in blood regeneration, contained a number of excellent tonic qualities, so it was not for me to say that the remedies mentioned were valueless.

By this time Maud, with her purchase still unfinished, was exasperated. "Will you *please* let me have a minute of his time?"

My response was to demand abruptly, "Vendor, how much do you want for that incense burner?"

Somewhat distracted from the main issue, he mentioned a price close to the real value and, after a protest or two, the final compromise was made. We stood there politely while he wrapped up the rest of his stock and muttered half to himself, "*Hsi chi deh hen!* How did this foreigner learn that my head is dizzy and my stomach hurts? Not even one word did I say—yet he knew. *Ai-ya!*"

As he bowed himself away, I told him, "Come to the dispensary tomorrow morning. I'll give you some foreign medicine for that *mao-ping* (disease)."

"Really, George," Maud would complain, "when you turn the front porch into an annex for the hospital, I think it's going too far."

"Well, your incense burner cost less than you expected, didn't it?"

"Naturally. You had the poor man so scared about his condition that he almost *gave* us the object."

"Then why the protest? Your purchase is satisfactory, and tomorrow he will be given treatment That ought to make everybody happy."

"This isn't by any chance a racket you're starting with those vendors, is it?"

"Tch! Tch! What a suspicious nature you're developing!" I answered, and hurried her toward our delayed meal.

The expression, "The whole world is my parish," credited to a famous divine, seems to apply peculiarly to the physician in any Oriental field. Pressed on all sides by the sick and afflicted, he soon finds himself offering medical advice as he would never dream of doing at home. Even the most rural Chinese have learned through the years the value of certain foreign drugs. When a Westerner, regardless of profession, takes to the road, he is surrounded at every village halt by country people asking for a little iodine or quinine or Epsom salts for their respective difficulties. The physician soon begins to consider the entire population his special field for practice: an assumption that sometimes leads to ludicrous complications.

On a street corner close to the hospital was a middle-aged beggar whose rags revealed filthy leg sores. One day as I halted beside this pitiable object, I decided that without a great deal of effort on our part we could put him on the path to health and decent living. To the usual whine for a copper, he was adding real tears, and conscious that no time was better than the present in which to do "*hao si*" (good deeds), I said, "You come with me! I have a little plan."

Tears and distorted expression gave place instantly to a look of calculation. Without a word, he caught up the wooden begging-bowl and followed.

In the dispensary I ordered the affected parts bathed thoroughly and treated. After this he was given a clean cotton jacket and told to return in two days. For a week or so I forgot the fellow completely, then seeing him one morning in his customary spot, I asked, "Did you go again to the dispensary?"

He mumbled some sort of reply as I noted that the sores seemed in even worse condition than before. This was more difficult to explain than the absence of the blue cotton jacket. Poor wretch, I thought, he may have sold the coat for food. "You shall go with me now," was my immediate decision.

This day he seemed much less willing to co-operate, but was finally persuaded to do so and received the same treatment as on the previous occasion, though without the gift of a jacket.

The third time I hauled him into the clinic, and "hauled" was literally the way it was accomplished. I said to Doctor Tu, "That is a queer case. Instead of reacting favorably to treatment, these sores get worse."

"They'll never be any better, *Beh Ih-seng*," Tu answered flatly.

"Why not? There's nothing malignant about them. The fellow seems to use some red medicine of his own —did you notice that?"

"Yes, I noticed." Then he added expressively, "You can no more cure that case, Doctor, than you can escape your own shadow in the sun."

This called for an explanation, and Tu gave it. I was still new to the city then and knew nothing of the business-like system under which this tribe of scarecrows preyed upon hard-working Chungkingese. Each beggar had some special affliction or deformity as his stock in trade for appealing to the sympathy of passersby. This man's was the fairly simple one of sores. The first time I had told him to follow, he probably thought Fortune had elected him its favorite, for foreigners recently arrived were notoriously more generous than the Chinese, who had been forced to put up with beggar rapacity for centuries. Stolidly he had endured the surprising bath and treatment, both equally distasteful to him, in the hope that the end would bring satisfactory reward. Instead, he had received only a cotton jacket, which while clean, was also old.

Out on the street again, it had been necessary for him to invest in a red paste that would irritate the sores quickly. This was painful and expensive. Why he allowed himself to be dragged back a second and then a third time, I am not sure. His first optimism about reward had certainly died much earlier, and it may be that he was simply afraid to disobey so determined a foreign devil.

By now, doubtless a little desperate, he must have racked his brain to find some way of staving off my good intentions. These, of course, were continuing to cost him money and discomfort. The particular corner he claimed as his own was the one allotted him by the Beggars' Guild for the purpose of earning a living. He could go nowhere else without getting into trouble with them; on the other hand, if he remained, I would, in time, rob him of his special "appeal."

For months afterwards, on my approach, he got up hastily and lost himself in the crowd. But as time passed and I continued to let him alone, peace must have descended on his troubled soul. When I left Chungking, he still occupied that corner—rags and sores just as I had first seen them.

Later on, I was accidentally concerned with another beggar's plight of a much more tragic nature. One day I was passing the Catholic Cathedral with an American friend, when a young street arab missed his step on the stairs leading to the next level and hurtled to the bottom.

From where we stood on the upper thoroughfare, the child could be seen lying crushed on the flagstones, and I started at once down toward him. My companion instantly clutched my arm. "George," he begged, "for Heaven's sake don't get mixed up in that!"

"What are you talking about?" I returned indignantly. "If he's still alive, I may be able to do something."

"But there isn't one chance in a hundred that he is—you saw him fall. And whether he's dead or alive, if you go near him you'll probably bring more trouble on your own head and on the hospital than you ever expected to meet."

"That's a risk I'll have to run," I replied pulling my arm free.

My friend's shoulders shrugged expressively. "Well, I can't stop you, but you can be very certain of one thing: if you touch that boy, you assume full responsibility for his injuries, for the whole Beggars' Guild will swear that you killed him and will bring suit for compensation."

I halted in painful indecision as the crowd below closed in about the child's body. This was my first medical experience in having to choose between immediate need and eventual cost. Sober reality reminded me of the lawsuits that had already involved the foreign hospitals. Also, I remembered uncomfortably that my personal altercation with Colonel Chu had once exposed our own institution to danger. In the end, permitting wisdom rather than impulse to guide me, I turned away, though for some time afterward it

18

was hard to forget that once when a child might have needed my help this had not been offered.

On a number of occasions in Chungking I had been invited to attend a theatrical performance but had never found it convenient to accept. The opportunity came, finally, one afternoon when our host at an elaborate official feast suggested that we go on from there to a play. Long since familiar with the way Chinese hospitality devoured time, I had left word at the hospital not to count on me that evening, so I was free to follow inclination.

While we sat there in the official residence, finishing Eight Precious Pudding, cracking watermelon seeds between teeth, and sipping flower-scented tea, I asked questions about the Chinese drama.

The theater seems to have been first established in A.D. 735 during the reign of the Tang Emperor, Yuen Tsung. This ruler's favorite concubine was Yang Kuei-fei, famous in Chinese lore for her beauty and artful ways. Trying to plan some novel form of entertainment for the lady, the Son of Heaven conceived the idea of having attractive girls and boys trained to recite historical episodes. When this preparation was completed, the young actors and actresses, magnificently costumed, gave the first performance in an orchard pavilion, and from that original stage setting Chinese Thespians received their name, "Students of the Pear Garden."

An orchestra of several hundred musicians added to the affair, for in Yuen Tsung's time every educated person could play some instrument, and Yang Kuei-fei, herself, was supposed to have no mean ability with a lute. The first performance was madly acclaimed, and, on the wave of popularity, each succeeding presentation outdid the previous one in size and splendor. Rapidly becoming a synonym for extravagance, this newest art contributed toward the eventual downfall of the emperor and his irresistible lady.

In the reign that followed there was a sharp reversion to economy, and as a result dramatic exhibitions were banned throughout the kingdom for years. After its rebirth the drama progressed slowly. Limited as were all serious writers to the Confucian mediums of poetry, essays, and scholarly treatise, no one would stoop to creating plays for popular consumption.

Not until the Mongols (A.D. 1280—A.D. 1368), with their Tartar love of pageantry and entertainment, did the drama really come into its own. Six hundred years later, the Manchu Empress Dowager was to give the theater still another impetus by means of her own open enthusiasm for such performances.

During its periods of unpopularity, the theater acquired a disreputable name that continued with it even in prosperity. Girls were no longer permitted to appear on the stage, and men filled the roles for both sexes. Chinese, almost incredibly tolerant about many things, evidently made no allowances for the artistic temperament. Actors were considered a rowdy, unstable lot and so valueless to ordinary living that they were placed among the lowest groups in the social scale.

The early idea of using open pavilions continued through the centuries. Even in towns and cities theater buildings were slight, flimsy affairs; frequently the plays were given in open spaces such as temple courtyards. In the rural districts, when a troupe of players arrived, they were lucky to find even the crudest sort of shelter ready for them. Their presentations were most popular on village market days when the surrounding country-side might be expected to increase the size of the audience. All that was ever needed to set the scene was a background of silk draperies, for the Chinese actor depends entirely on costume for props, and the stage has neither scenery nor furniture.

When the plays are short, a whole series may be given in succession with the performance running for hours. The Chinese theatergoer not only demands but receives his money's worth.

The Chungking theater, like so many others inland, was a bamboo and mat shed with wooden boards laid on the ground for flooring. The lobby, nothing more than a large bare entrance, was crowded by friendly groups engaged in the sort of small talk one hears the world over in such places. Leading us inside to specially reserved seats at the front, the ushers tossed each of us a steaming hot towel to be used for refreshing hands and face. After being used, these were collected, only to be redistributed time and again during the evening.

From the very first we were the cynosure of all eyes, for our host was one of the most important men in the city, and several of his guests were also of the official class. The stage manager, having learned in advance of our contemplated arrival, was apparently prepared to pay these dignitaries full honor. He now came out on the platform to extend them a special welcome. After this had been courteously acknowledged, the show began, and we settled down to make ourselves as comfortable as possible on the customary narrow wooden benches.

Afterwards I learned that the setting was Southwest China, and that the plot dealt with a son's determination to wander abroad seeking fortune and with his family's equally strong resolve to keep him at home. As might have been expected, for Good always triumphs in the old Chinese drama, the son finally made the supreme sacrifice to filial duty and remained under the paternal rooftree.

Entirely new to such performances, I could never have figured out the whole story for myself, though the audience helped me to partial understanding. Informality was the keynote of this entertainment, and whenever any one of the spectators felt inclined to express himself about theme or action, he interrupted the

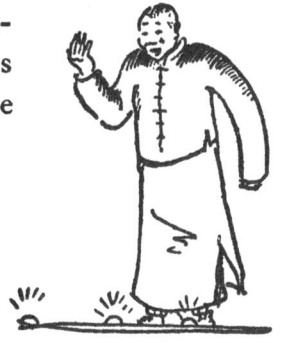

actors to do so. There were several hot arguments on the floor concerning the son's conflict between duty and desire. Needless to say, those in favor of filial obedience greatly outnumbered the others.

In spite of the uncomfortable seat, I was thoroughly enjoying this whole affair, for the audience was almost as interesting as the drama. Tea, fruit, and sweetmeats were being served constantly in response to orders bawled over the heads of the crowd. As people recognized friends, they rose to bow ceremoniously and exchange greetings; the fact that a play was in progress did not seem to bother anyone. Most of the time the din on the stage, probably designed to exceed the noises of the house, was terrific. Suddenly in a lull, I heard someone call out, "That's *Beh Ih-seng* with those officials."

"Who?" another several rows away yelled back.

"*Beh Ih-seng* at the American hospital. That one who won't permit spitting on the floors."

My ears grew hot as one gaze after another sought me out. Unfortunately, my host had heard this byplay as well as I. He now rose and leaned over me, indicating that I must stand and bow to the audience. I complied much like a puppet on a string, and from all over the room this courtesy was returned.

Attempting, after this unexpected limelight, to sink back into the protecting shadows of my distinguished sponsors, I felt sure that the evening's excitement had reached its peak. However, just as the audience seemed to have forgotten us for other interests, one of the actors, in swinging his sword, struck a companion accidentally, and the injured player fell to the floor.

A moment only was the action of the drama halted, then after brief discussion the management evidently decided that "the play must go on." The troupe took up positions a little away from the casualty, and the performance was resumed.

At this point my host sent for the manager and, without consulting me, magnanimously offered my services in the emergency. "I myself will go up on the stage with you, *Beh Ih-seng*," he assured me.

"I shall be glad to look at that man, but not on the stage," I insisted, having already been sufficiently conspicuous for one evening.

"But, *Beh Ih-seng*, the audience will want to watch you."

"Your Excellency, both the wounded player and I will be *puh hao ee si* (embarrassed) to have so many people looking at us."

He smiled benignantly. "*Beh Ih-seng* is too modest, and he does not know actors! Moreover, the audience has paid to see everything that happens in this theater and your heart, Doctor, is too kind to deprive them of this."

In the end I went up on the stage with him and there took care of the patient, whose condition, a slight concussion, left me to be *puh hao ee si* all by myself. There was little else wrong with the man. After bandaging the wound with a proffered towel and ordering him removed to a quiet place for rest, I was ready to return to my seat.

Again I reckoned without my host, whom the audience seemed to be bombarding with questions. He now turned graciously to me and said, "*Beh Ih-seng*, you have been asked to grant a great favor to all these citizens of Chungking. They are very much interested in learning about foreign medicine and will be most grateful if you will tell them about it."

"Perhaps when the play is finished," I protested feebly, waving toward the dramatic performance that was still in progress.

"Unimportant! That will continue for sometime, and the audience wishes you to speak now." Thus easily dismissing the major show, he ushered me to the front of the stage. Since I was not equipped with a megaphone, it was a physical impossibility for those at the rear of the building to hear me above the actors' noises. To overcome this hindrance, whole rows of them now came forward and a number climbed up on the stage around me.

My first annoyance disappeared as I recognized an unusual opportunity to publicize the hospital's work, and for a solid half hour I talked. The crowd was paying close attention, and I might have continued indefinitely but for the fact that the play had come to a halt. The actors, thoroughly disgruntled over having lost their audience, were standing about in groups muttering to themselves. Suddenly conscious that I was the cause of all the dissatisfaction, I brought my speech to an abrupt end.

The manager rushed forward to thank me, and from all over the building came voluble expressions of appreciation. This ovation merely added fuel to the flame of displeasure on the stage and the actors' remarks grew louder and more insulting. Again the manager assumed charge—this must have been one of the busiest evenings in his whole career. He explained to his players that but for my assistance, one of their members might now be dead, which was certainly stretching the truth in my favor, then demanded that they apologize over a bowl of tea. There on the stage the calming beverage was served to all, and, between sips, the disaffected Thespians and I ended competition for the spotlight once and for all.

By this time, as might be imagined, I was more than ready to go home, but when we returned to our seats, ushers brought us an elaborate supper on trays. This repast, which had been previously ordered by his Excellency, lasted for another fifty-five minutes.

When departure was finally made, after six hours in the theater, the performance was still continuing, and the rest of the audience showed no signs of leaving.

I realized afresh that the Chinese were certainly made of sterner stuff than Americans, for my first theatrical entertainment in Chungking had left me more exhausted than if I had been through a long, hard day at the hospital.

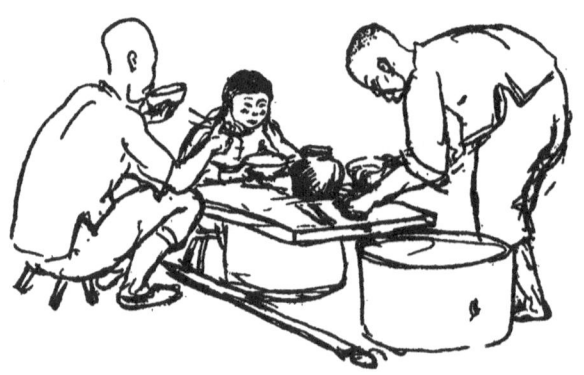

CHAPTER XVIII

I Promise a Son

The Chinese sense of humor is broad and deep, but two subjects—posterity and filial piety—are rarely permitted to come within its bounds. For the individual to become facetious about either of these is not only ill-advised but dangerous, as I discovered from as harrowing an experience as I have ever known before or since.

One morning bright and early, a Colonel T'sen came to my private office, and on being told by the clerk that I would be in the operating room for another two hours, he sat down to wait for my return. I seem for some reason to have been allergic to colonels, for all of my real military difficulties in Chungking began and ended with that rank. This worthy, however, was much more important than his title might have led one to expect. He was a favorite with General Den, the war-lord, and had been temporarily placed in active military control of the city while Den was away dipping his fingers in a political pie to the Southwest.

When I finally appeared and was told how long this visitor had been waiting, I realized that something serious was afoot. The average Chinese has all the time in the world but this was not true, naturally, of officials and militarists; in their affairs it was always the other fellow who was forced to cool his heels. In spite of the delay, he was surprisingly pleasant, and contrary to Chinese fashion, came straight to the point. His first four wives, he informed me, had proved most disappointing in presenting him with seven girls between them and not a single son. Several months earlier he had taken a fifth wife, a girl from a family with the reputation for strong and prolific women, and she was now entering the fourth month of pregnancy. Someone had told him that foreign hospitals were unusually successful in caring for prospective mothers and in safely delivering their babies; to arrange such treatment for his own wife he had come here this morning.

During the conversation he made a number of references to the importance of this infant's being a boy, but I thought little of that; all Chinese express themselves similarly about an expected child. We discussed arrangements; then promising to bring his wife in that very day for an examination, he rose to go. "It is said foreign doctors have much more skill in these matters than do Chinese," he remarked with a smile at parting. "I am depending on you, *Beh Ih-seng*, to see that my child is a boy."

"Lay down your heart, Colonel," I returned carelessly, "we'll have to see what can be done in this matter."

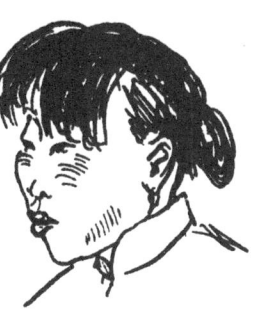

Several hours later he returned with his wife. The girl was dignified, well-bred, and extremely intelligent, and I wondered what evil fortune had persuaded her family to let her become the fifth wife to this militarist, a far from enviable rank in any household. Was it possible that the Colonel had claimed her as a prize of war in some foray of the past year? I was not likely ever to know her story, but even in that first interview I hoped compassionately that this child might be a son and raise her status in the household. That later on I should be wishing the same thing much more fervently for my own sake, I did not then realize. Examination showed her in excellent condition, and after careful instructions to which she listened most attentively, I told them to return in three weeks.

At the appointed time they did so, accompanied on this occasion by the Colonel's special bodyguard of twenty soldiers, his four other wives, and several men and women.

I protested politely that the hospital could not permit entrance to all these people for a patient's routine visit.

My heretofore suave Colonel turned suddenly severe, "These are all members of our family; the birth of this child is of great importance to them. When my wife comes here to stay, many of our relatives from beyond Chungking will come also. I shall wish rooms for them in the hospital."

"A hospital, Colonel T'sen," I explained, "is not like an inn; it cares for sick people only. Your wife, as patient, will be accommodated in this building; all others in your party must stay elsewhere."

For a moment or two he continued the argument, then abruptly terminated it with, "*Ko ee!* (Can do)."

It seemed perfectly natural for him to accept the situation agreeably. While he occupied his present position as Den's representative, more than one Chung-kingese politician would be glad to entertain members of the Colonel's family for as long as they cared to stay in the city. That he had hoped to make an unprecedentedly handsome gesture of hospitality by chartering the foreign institution for the celebration did not occur to me until later, nor did I dream that his acceptance of my alternative was due simply to fear of antagonizing me, and through me, the supernatural forces involved in arranging for his heir.

At regular periods he brought the young wife in for routine examination, and on each of these occasions at parting, reminded me pleasantly, "Remember, *Beh Ih-seng*, I am depending on you for a son."

I would reply as genially, "Yes, yes, I remember."

Almost five months of prenatal care passed; then one morning R——, my closest friend in the Methodist Compound, stepped into my office, carefully closed the door, and asked gravely, "George, how did all this talk get started about your promising Colonel T'sen a son?"

"I don't know what you mean by 'all this talk.' The Colonel and I have had a little joke between us ever since he first asked me to take care of his wife."

"Well, you may think it's a joke, but I can tell you right now the Colonel doesn't. He's deadly serious about the whole thing."

"Nonsense! The Colonel is nobody's fool. He has sense enough to know that nobody can do anything about changing the sex of a child."

R—— shook his head. "You ought to realize by this time that there isn't any abracadabra the Chinese cannot accept on the subject of birth, particularly in the field of foreign medicine, about which they know so little. Take my advice and lose no time making Colonel T'sen understand that you personally are helpless about influencing things one way or the other."

On the very next visit when the Colonel made his usual reference to a son, I said, "I certainly hope your wish comes true, but of course, you understand that no one under Heaven has any power to regulate such matters."

The patient's startled glance flew to my face then dropped as swiftly to the floor, while her husband declared with a short laugh, "You jest, Doctor, is it not so?"

"Of course not. I am doing everything possible to help your wife bear a strong child, and for both your sakes, I hope it will be a son. More than that I cannot promise."

Colonel T'sen stepped a little closer. His eyes had narrowed to slits and his voice had a steely edge. "For five months you have promised me a son, Doctor, and I have made all my arrangements for one. There must be no mistake about this!"

Before I could make a satisfactory retort, he bowed and left the office with his wife following, Chinese fashion, sedately in his steps.

It still seemed incredible that the Colonel believed I could control this matter, but that was exactly what he did. This time it was I who hunted up R——. "You know, you were right about that fellow," I confessed. "He made it very clear that I am supposed to deliver the goods according to his order."

R—— looked worried. "I was afraid of that. Rumor says he plans to spend several thousand dollars (Mexican) on feasting and entertaining. A number of relatives from upcountry have already arrived in Chungking, and others are adding to their numbers daily. I don't mean to be a calamity howler, but you're in a dangerous position. If the infant should be a girl, the Colonel not only loses a lot of money—he loses 'face,' for he has advertised widely that this child will be a son. To have to admit failure of his plans—well, he's not the type to take his punishment lying down; you know that as well as I."

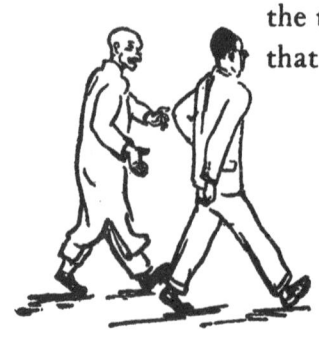

"What do you think he'll do?"

"I wish I could guess. So far as armed force is concerned, he's the most powerful man in Chungking today; and as long as Den is absent, the Colonel is answerable only to himself."

"Perhaps General Den will return before the affair takes place."

"I doubt if he or any of your other friends among the officials would interfere in this instance. You know how the Chinese feel about a promise, and when it has to do with a man's son, the matter becomes a grave one."

"But I tell you there was never any real promise; his statements and mine were always accompanied by laughter!"

"I'll bet the laughter on his part wasn't very hearty. Do you know what I'd do?" he asked abruptly, and answered the question in the same breath, "I think I'd run."

"What do you mean?"

"Have sudden business somewhere else in China and ask one of the other foreign doctors who's unhampered by past conversations with the husband to look after her."

"But she's my patient and a good one. My only promise in this affair was made to myself to see her through safely, and I intend to do just that."

"Even if you wreck the hospital work?"
19

"But that's absurd!"

"All right! Suppose you talk it over with your friend Strobel and two or three others. See what they advise."

Hourly I felt more of a fool, but I did what R—— suggested about sounding out others.

To my astonishment they agreed that urgent business elsewhere was the wisest procedure. I was reminded that in dangerous moments the Chinese themselves always considered retreat the best possible strategy.

"You mean," I asked one of them sharply, "that I am to desert a patient and, incidentally, lose my own self-respect on the chance that this militarist may make things hot? Anyway, who can say the child won't be a boy?"

"Can you say it will? If it shouldn't be, you stand a chance of losing a good deal more than self-respect."

I was by this time completely at a loss what to do. Finally, when the event was two weeks off, I told the Colonel that I had business at the Rockefeller Hospital in Pieping (true enough) and that I might have to be leaving in a day or two. I would make every arrangement for his wife's care, however, and one of the other foreign doctors would look after her.

All but the first part of this announcement seemed to fall on deaf ears. "If *Beh Ih-seng* will tell me when he expects to leave, my wife and I and our closest relatives will go down river also on the same steamer.

We trust no one but *Beh Ih-seng* to manage this important affair."

"I'll be glad to let you know, if I have to go, Colonel T'sen," I managed to reply, recognizing that my adversary had promptly outbluffed me. Once and for all, the idea of eluding responsibility for this affair was settled; and though I was just where I had started, my mind felt better about the whole affair.

A week in advance the patient entered the hospital. She seemed in excellent physical shape and was, as she had always been, pleasantly co-operative. Her presence however, did nothing to boost my natural buoyancy. Every time I passed her door I thought with grim realism, "Well, Number Five, you and I sink or swim together!"

The carefully reckoned day on which the child was expected to arrive dawned bright and clear, in sharp contrast to Chungking's usual gray winter mist. This seemed such a good omen that my spirits rose for the first time in weeks. The stimulation, however, was short lived, for the hours dragged by without a sign of activity.

The Colonel with his host of relatives plied me and the staff endlessly with questions, and our repeated answers that Nature took her own time about such things left them unsatisfied.

For five days this continued. With an army camped on our doorstep there was no escape even for a moment. Every time I glanced out a window I saw more of the

T'sen cohorts impatiently striding up and down the hospital walks. Opening my office door, I was at once besieged by troops and relatives swarming in the corridors. When I managed to slip over to our residence, the most importunate of these kept at my heels all the way. In the house Maud greeted me with a forced smile that in no way hid her fears. The hospital routine was becoming completely disorganized; hurrying about its duties, the staff cast nervous glances to right and left and jumped whenever anyone spoke above a whisper. Personally, I had reached the place where I could see myself walking down the road to lunacy and could not lift a finger to check the advance.

On the sixth day the siege was broken by the patient's showing signs of progress. At once Colonel, relatives, and troops, being assured of action, settled down to a period of pleasant waiting. Needless to say, my own nerves received no such soporific. Having felt that nothing could be worse than the days of inactivity, I could now, so close to the hour of sentence, look back on them as almost carefree.

To my surprise the girl, in spite of apparent good condition, showed every sign of having a long, hard period of labor, and, under pressure of work, my own worries took a second place. Twelve, eighteen, twenty-four hours passed, and the patient, who until this time had conducted herself admirably, now succumbed to hysteria. In my opinion, sedatives for the mother carried

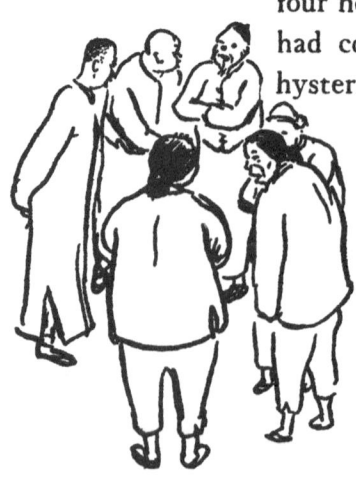

too great risk for the child, and by the time another twelve hours of strain had passed, I decided to operate.

The Colonel offered no objections when I told him of the need for this, but immediately he and twenty-odd uniformed men pushed into the operating room to occupy the section usually filled by students, and to watch every move I made. There was a great deal of chatter from that quarter until the patient's groans quieted under anesthesia. Her sudden silence seemed to be contagious, for after that one could have heard a pin drop. Whatever my own mental state, there was no slightest doubt that each spectator was having the opportunity of his life in watching this foreign operation.

I performed an episiotomy and used forceps on the baby's head. Slowly but surely the child fought its way into the world. The closer it came, the more frightened I grew. Never before in my life had I prayed about an infant's sex, but I did so then. When I discovered that the Colonel had been given a son, I almost dropped the baby.

Colonel and bodyguard now came down from their box seats. "What is it? What is it?" they called out one after the other.

It was all I could do to answer, "A boy!" Giving the baby over to a nurse, I turned again to my patient.

The young mother was in a critical condition, and as I worked on her, I heard the nurse call to me for help. I glanced around at the commotion. To my horror, the Colonel had taken the newborn child in his arms and was passing it from one officer friend to the other. When he caught my eye, he called out, "Come with us, Doctor! We go now to show the child to family and friends!"

Abruptly I found emotional vent for all the anxiety experienced in the weeks past. "Colonel T'sen," I shouted, "I have seen your son safely into the world; if you choose now to kill it, that is your affair. If you wish it to live, give the child at once to the nurse; and don't speak to me again until your wife has had proper care!"

I turned again to my patient. That anyone had dared thus to insult him before his brother officers must have taken his breath away, but he got over it quickly enough, for when I had a chance to look up, I noticed that the nurse was once more in possession of the baby. By the time it had been given the usual routine treatment after birth, I called out that the father might have it for a moment, and saw them march into the hall. The mother was now ready to be wheeled back to her room. When I decided nothing further could be done for her at the moment, I left a nurse in charge and joined the general assembly.

It was fortunate that the hospital held no desperately ill patients, for bedlam reigned. When I appeared, the proud father insisted on introducing me to the crowd, all of whom I had met far too often in the past weeks ever to enjoy seeing them again. He followed this by a speech in which I was thanked in flowery terms for my part in the affair. When these painful compliments came to an end, I replied briefly, then told him that the baby must now have peace and quiet. "Also," I added, "if you wish us to look after your son for a while, there must be no more visitors. Already he has been exposed to a variety of germs, and I fear for the child's safety."

For a moment the talk of germs left him a little dazed, then with usual vigor he protested, "But some of the family are not here this morning; it suits them better to come this afternoon."

I was adamant. "Either no more visitors or you may take the child home with you now."

The Colonel looked from one to the other of the group crowded about us. "*Muh iu fa tz!*" he conceded agreeably. "*Beh Ih-seng* has kept his promise that I would have a son; now we must do as he says."

Again the child was handed to the nurse, and as I finished giving her directions for the care of the infant, Colonel T'sen turned, again expressed his appreciation for my services, and concluded, "Truly the foreign doctors know much more about arranging for sons than do the Chinese."

"Long ago I told you that no man can control such things."

He laughed tolerantly. "You are much too humble, *Beh Ih-seng*. Now, where do you want your things?"

"What things?"

"Some little gifts for you."

I responded with the usual, "Most unworthy!" Chinese patients always gave doctors and nurses gifts when discharged from the hospital; that he was choosing to present his in advance was quite all right with me. "If you will be good enough to send them to my home, that will be best; at present, I must go look after other patients."

I slipped into the office, wrote a hasty note to Maud with the good news, and started rounds with a lighter heart than for a long, long time. The note proved unnecessary, for my wife in the short time that had transpired had already received the word from our servants and those in neighboring compounds and from a number of outside Chinese acquaintances as well. Later in the day she sent me one. It read, "For mercy's sake come home and explain what's going on here."

When I arrived, I found our entrance and yard crowded by coolies hovering over a mass of boxes and baskets. Sighting me, all smiled broadly. The gateman hurried to explain, "Gifts for *Beh Ih-seng* for giving Colonel T'sen a son."

Maud met me on the porch. "These bearers say they are from Colonel T'sen, and they insist that all of their loads are for us. There must be a mistake somewhere."

Questioning proved that the loads were all meant for our household. They were eventually deposited on the porch, and after I had given each coolie *t'sa chien* (tea money—a tip), the bearers sauntered happily down the walk, their carrying-poles and ropes now dangling from horny hands.

Maud and the servants were already peeking into containers, and when everything was finally unpacked, we found ourselves in possession of rolls of Chengtu silk and Suifu pongee, strips of handsome embroidery, painted silk scrolls, brasses, soapstone ornaments, and most incongruously, a number of cases of canned fruit from America. These last were not only hard to get in Chungking but were extremely expensive, and for a foreign household to fall heir to so many at once seemed like coming into a fortune. Many of these were cherries, my favorite fruit, a matter on which one of the Colonel's servants had carefully questioned our cook.

Colonel T'sen had been grimly determined to have a son, but typically Chinese, he had also been willing to pay well for what he got. In two weeks when the mother and baby were carried triumphantly home, he turned in the usual fees, then added an extra gift to the hospital treasury. When I considered these, I did not linger on the thought that but for a whim of Nature, things might have been very different.

My local mail now increased by leaps and bounds and in time came from provinces at the other end of

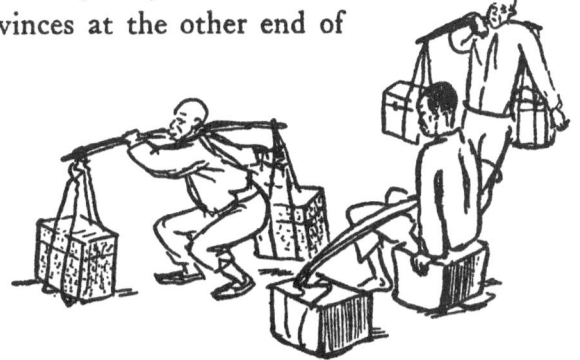

China. These letters, always on the same subject, were sent by prosperous husbands who stated that their wives were pregnant, and begged me to name my price for arranging the arrival of a son instead of a daughter. The futility of trying to explain that I had no influence in such matters was immediately apparent. All the evidence was against me—Colonel T'sen had a son, and how he had gotten it everybody seemed to know. I sent out a form answer to the effect that I was much too busy at the hospital to take any more obstetrical cases save ordinary ones. As I sat and wrote these amazing documents, I seemed to feel Chungking leaning over my shoulder like some old crone who was enjoying the moment to the full. In my ears her derisive cackles echoed for a long time afterward.

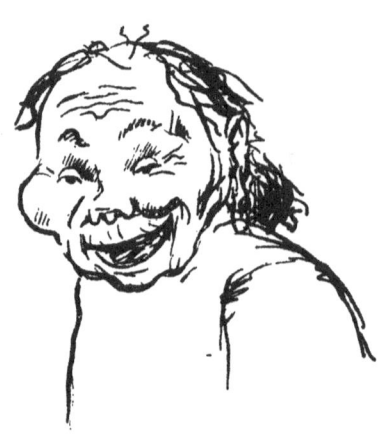

CHAPTER XIX

Tapping a Monkey's Brains

My wife had never been able to adapt herself physically to the Chungking climate. Doctor Strobel was now insisting on her immediate return to America, and since I could not accompany them, it seemed wiser for her to take the baby and go before she became too ill to travel alone. On the date finally decided upon I saw my family off on the steamer, and went back to a house that seemed to shout its emptiness when I entered the door.

Parnell was still with me, and we invited a new business man in port, named Harding, to share in our housekeeping arrangements. He was a cheerful soul with a magnificent voice, and in the mornings his jubilant notes would pull the plaster right off the bathroom ceiling.

On the surface life went much the same as usual. Most of my time was spent in the hospital; when at home, I had little responsibility, for the servants were entirely familiar with routine arrangements and needed only to be checked on such things as water filtering and food washing.

287

The cook, as was customary, did all the marketing. Occasionally when the word got around that some steamer steward was willing to part with a staple on which he had overstocked, I would hurry down a request. On one such occasion, I asked for a half dozen containers of ketchup. These were to be delivered to the water-front office of a business friend, whose coolies would bring the stuff to me on their next trip in our direction.

A few days later when I went home to dinner, the gateman handed me a note. It was from the friend who had received the ketchup consignment for me, and it read as follows:

Dear George:

You've always said you liked ketchup, and before heaven I believe it. It took three coolies to get this up to you. What in thunder are you going to do with it—take a beauty bath?

E.

As I walked nonchalantly to the pantry, I thought, My! E—— must have been feeling facetious when he wrote that—it seems like a lot of fuss to make over a half dozen bottles of ketchup. I swung open the door and stood there, suddenly weak from shock. On the floor arranged neatly in a row against the wall sat six five-gallon tins of ketchup. Before I could recover from the first blow, the attached bill met my eye and that finished the job.

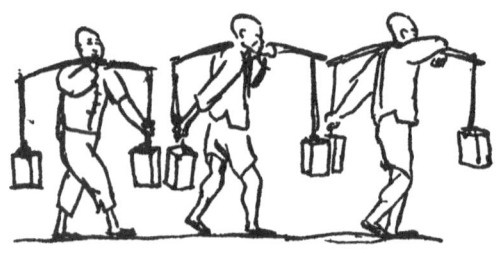

Stuck with thirty gallons of ketchup, I was determined to make good use of it. Morning, noon, and night a generous portion appeared on the table. Parnell and Harding, each of whom was more than ordinarily tough, I'd say, soon reached the place where their countenances assumed a sickly cast whenever the table-boy urged this delicacy upon them. Even I gradually lost all interest in piquant sauces made from the lowly tomato, and I have to confess I have never since entirely regained my first early enthusiasm for them.

One winter's afternoon just before dusk, I received a "hurry" call from a near-by mission. One of their oldest workers, a woman who had whole-heartedly devoted her life to Chungking, had been set ablaze by the explosion of an alcohol lamp. I rushed over but it was already too late to save her. Helpers had beaten out the flames, though not before her body was covered with third-degree burns. Death came shortly, and in this case was, I felt, a merciful release in more ways than one. She would soon have reached retirement age, and whenever I had talked with her in the past year, this fact which would necessitate her leaving China to live at home was always uppermost in the conversation. This was a paramount fear with many foreigners, men and women alike; when people have invested their lives in a country and its inhabitants, they usually want to remain there for the rest of their days.

This was especially true in the case of the burned woman, since her life for many years had been predominantly Chinese in interest and sympathy. There is a saying to the effect that China always passively assimilates her conquerors; she does something equally subtle to her friends. Of all the Americans and Europeans who have ever lived in Cathay, those who have actively disliked the land and its people are proportionately few. In time many foreigners become more pro-Chinese than the Chinese themselves. It was always fascinating for me to watch the antipathy of new arrivals change to judicious interest and then to enthusiastic liking for I, myself, was a standard example of this process.

However tragic at the last, this particular woman's life had ended on this soil she loved; and it would have pleased her to know that Chinese from all over the province came into Chungking to pay tribute to her memory. The completeness with which she had merged her own identity with theirs I think they realized no more than the foreigners did until the day of the funeral. Then all of us received a real shock. In her will careful directions had been given regarding the funeral; she wished a Christian service at the church, but after that everything was to be done in Chinese fashion. This ended, of course, with a typical funeral procession of wailing mourners dressed in white, winding in and out the miles of narrow streets that lay between the church and the cemetery. For the first time Chungking had the experience of watching East and West mingle customs and traditions around the sacrament of death.

As the months of Maud's absence passed, I found myself torn between two interests—my family and the work. Against my own medical judgment I tried to convince myself that all my wife needed was a short furlough in her native land. With strength restored she could then return to Chungking and we could continue as originally planned. It was Strobel, of course, who made me see that the fascination of the work was leading me toward wishful thinking and away from reality. There was no reason to believe that Maud would ever be able to live in the Chungking, and the wisest plan for all concerned was for me to join her at home.

As I was gradually arriving at this conclusion, my wife began to exert pressure from her end of the line. At eighty-eight cents a word she now indulged in a series of cables and sent them collect. Her style in these was almost as expansive as if they were traveling under five-cent postage. She told me in detail of her improvement and of the baby's progress, inquired solicitously about my own health and signed herself thoughtfully, "With love."

After paying for a half dozen lengthy messages, I grew desperate and cabled back. "Use Board of Foreign Missions code."

This move was not so wise as it had first seemed. The next cable from Maryland came in code. It contained the information that Maud was ill with acute nephritis and the doctor said there was little hope.

This time I forgot cost and, throwing discretion to the winds, cabled back, "More details of your condition."

By return came the answer: "Sorry, I got the code mixed up. Father has nephritis, not I. When are you coming home? Love from both of us."

I was by now emotionally as well as financially close to bankruptcy. I sat down at once and wrote my request to the Board for a successor.

When the word spread about Chungking that I was leaving, questions came thick and fast. Chinese have always used the diplomatic excuses of sickness or family trouble to explain resignation from public positions. When I offered my wife's ill health as reason for my own departure, none of the Chinese believed it the real one. It was inconceivable that a man would permit his wife's physical condition to uproot him from his work; all over the world Chinese were pursuing careers while their wives and families remained at home.

Since my progress in the Chungking medical field seemed satisfactory, where did the trouble lie, they wanted to know? One of my closest friends in the city, Tang, an official high in the Customs Service, asked me with unusual directness, "What is the real difficulty, Doctor?"

"You mean the name of Mrs. Basil's illness?"

"No, why are you leaving?"

I explained that, strange as it might seem, my wife's inability to live in Chungking was the only reason.

He let the subject drop and passed easily into a discussion of the growing friendliness between Szechuen and the Nanking Government. When this had been considered in every phase, he asked slowly, "If I form a committee of business men to build a good private hospital, Doctor, will you be its superintendent?"

I expressed my appreciation then added, "If I might remain in Chungking, Tang, I'd stay right in this institution."

"You are happy in the hospital—is the city perhaps at fault?"

"Neither hospital nor city! I would rather work in Chungking than anywhere else on earth."

He did not speak of the subject again, but each year since my return to America a letter has come from Tang saying, "When you are ready to become the superintendent, your hospital will be built."

Today I am inclined to be glad that money and effort never went into an enterprise that seems above all others to hold a fatal attraction for Japanese bombers.

Whenever a friend undertakes a journey, the Chinese speed him on his way with novel entertainments. Tang gave me a dinner at Chungking's newest edifice—a night club. The decorations were imitative of such

20

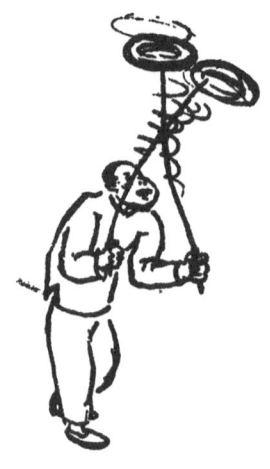

places the world over. Tables were set along the walls under dim lights; there was an orchestra, floor space for dancing, and to my astonishment, young Chinese women as dancing partners at so much a ticket. This was Western innovation with a vengeance, and I wondered how some of the older Chinese guests at the other tables were going to react to this Western form of recreation. In the port cities old-fashioned Chinese have of necessity become used to seeing their sons and daughters adopt foreign ballroom dancing, a "barbarism" they can never condone. But Chungking, so far inland, had seemed safe from such inroads on propriety, and I wondered if the owner of this establishment had not perhaps invested his money unwisely.

After the usual feast of many courses, the floor show began. Much of this was typically Chinese, musicians, tumblers, and jugglers filling most of the program. Girls appeared to sing, but that was all. There were perhaps twenty guests at our table—the only foreigners, Parnell, Harding, and I. Tang presented each of us with a string of tickets for the dancing, and I noticed with interest that the girls seemed none too anxious to have partners. When they could not evade the issue, they much preferred the men of their own race to the three of us. Most of the other patrons sat watching with set smiles on their faces; others concentrated on food and kept their eyes averted from the shocking spectacle of mixed dancing. Chungking, it was evident, had not become so modern as she wished to believe.

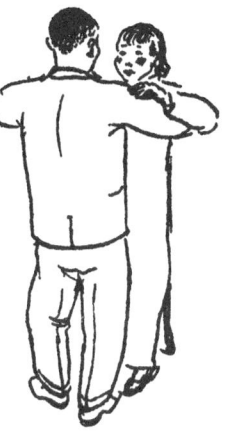

The most elaborate feast I attended was given by a group of forty civic leaders. I was the only foreigner present, and my host told me in advance that I might expect some surprises. They wanted me to remember this particular feast, and they went to unlimited trouble to have dishes that were not only rare but that belonged, in some instances, to tradition rather than popular usage. I had attended my full share of feasts in Chungking and had always enjoyed the good food thoroughly; this, however, was unlike anything I had yet experienced, and if I live to be Methusaleh's age, I shall not forget the details.

Before I left home I realized that as guest of honor, I would have to partake of everything on the menu before anyone else did. There was certain to be a good deal of hot wine served, and I prepared for this emergency by drinking several ounces of olive oil.

Alcohol loses its potency in the presence of olive oil; it does, though, have one unpleasant effect: in belching, which is the sign of appreciation for Chinese food and must find expression again and again during a meal, this mixture is quite likely to make one blow soap bubbles.

As I had expected, the wine was served soon after my arrival, and with it came several singsong girls. It was suggested that we play the popular finger game for drinks with each of these charmers. This pastime, without the refreshments, I had learned years before from "Navy Juniors," and most American schoolboys are familiar with it.

Each player throws forward his hands in one of three positions. The first, a doubled fist, symbolizes rock; the second, an open palm—paper; the third, two outstretched fingers—scissors. The throwing is simultaneous, and the penalty for losing is another drink.

If the combination is two fingers and a closed fist, the two-finger position loses, for scissors cannot cut rock. On the other hand, they win over a flat palm, for scissors can cut paper; and a flat palm wins over closed fist, for paper can cover rock. The Chinese use this and a half dozen other such games at all their feasts. The wine, however, is served in minute cups, and while heating increases its potency, the amount consumed rarely causes drunkenness. Intemperate drinking is not a Chinese weakness; the national vice is gambling.

After the first try or two, the girls faded from the scene; the men kept it up only a little longer, then the feast proceeded in earnest.

While we sat nibbling the ubiquitous watermelon seeds, a whole roast pig was brought in. I was invited to take the first piece, but found this difficult with no carving implements except chopsticks, so I asked for a kitchen knife. When this arrived, it was suggested that I cut my piece from the forehead, which was considered the choicest spot, though I never knew why, for when I complied and placed this morsel in my mouth, I found it too tough to swallow.

When everyone had eaten of the pig, bowls of soup were served. This was, of course, delicious. It was followed by flaky rice with the second meat delicacy.

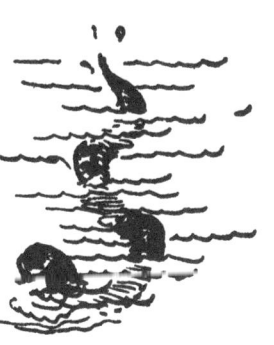

Boned chicken appeared next and was succeeded by what seemed to be eel. My first thought was, "This is the only time I've ever seen eel served at a Chinese feast." When I mentioned this to the neighbor on my right, he said, "This is a rare water snake, Doctor. It is hard to get and very expensive."

I lost my appetite for the article, though foolishly so, for there was little difference, as far as I could see, between eel and water snake; and now that our Southwest offers rattlesnakes as edible, my squeamishness on that occasion seems doubly absurd.

Shark fins were now served, common enough at any first-rate Chinese feast, and after these a dish of tiny, slender legs somewhat like a squab's. The flavor was different, however, and after eating several, I commented, "These are the best frog's legs I have ever tasted."

The guest on the right again came to the rescue with an explanation. They were, he told me, the legs of white rats. These, specially bred, raised, and fed on vegetables and grains are considered a delicacy much to be preferred to wild rodents like squirrels and rabbits. I thought afterwards that taste depends upon the point of view, for in America we eat these other members of the same family without giving them a thought.

Water chestnuts, bamboo sprouts, mushrooms, all made their appearance and were enjoyed to the full.

A servant now placed before me a bowl of shrimp, removed from the shells but still alive. When I first saw these small pink creatures moving about, I was afraid the olive oil had failed in its work. My hosts invited me to take the first one, and after a good deal of difficulty I got this between the chopsticks. I had the feeling that it would never make the trip from the bowl to my mouth so I threw it at myself and missed. The second time I caught it between my lips, clamped down and held it. This was a mistake, for the creature found time to wriggle. I swallowed hastily, and it wriggled all the way down. I grabbed my wine cup and gulped hastily in the hope of anesthetizing the shrimp. The method worked. I managed to get two more down in this way and would have had no trouble, could I have brought myself to chew them, as did the Chinese, who are as fond of raw shrimp as most Americans are of raw oysters.

The dishes continued to come: rice bowls were constantly refilled, and then toward the last, the *piece de résistance* arrived. The servants carried in a small table unlike anything I had ever seen before. In the center

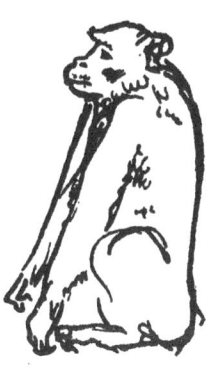

of the top was a hole perhaps six inches in diameter and beneath this a shelf on which a small, live monkey was chained. When one of the men came over and presented me with a short-handled mallet, I asked what I was supposed to do with it. It was explained that in olden times, doctors had considered it of marvelous benefit for a man to partake of this breed of monkey's brains. The servants would now fasten the monkey's head in the hole at the top, and with the mallet I was to crack the skull and take the first spoonful of brains. The Chinese, as a race, are so busy looking after their humankind that they waste little sentiment on animals. While I had done my share of hunting in years past, to stand there and kill a poor, helpless monkey that had not the slightest chance of escape was one of the most distasteful propositions I had ever faced.

I tried to beg off, but they insisted that, being a doctor, I knew where the brains were located better than anyone else. There seemed nothing to do but grant their request. I gritted my teeth, took a good aim, and with one blow the monkey died. Whatever contribution this luckless simian's brains may have made to his alleged human relatives is a problem yet to be solved; at least Chinese tradition was duly served, and the American present registered another unique experience.

In spite of the exotic menu which must have cost a small fortune—the monkey, I learned afterwards, was brought by special messenger all the way from Southwest Yunnan—the conversation at that feast was extremely interesting and modern. The men present were either city officials or army officers, and they were extremely anxious about further promotion of the commercial airplane service that was already operating between the coast and Chungking. In 1930, returning to Szechuen after having escorted a desperately ill patient to the coast, I had traveled by plane as far as Hankow. Many of these men present had covered the whole distance by air so that they knew from personal experience the convenience of this new service.

I can remember that once during the evening a reference was made to Den's military demonstration in which the bomb had been dropped on the crowd, and memory made me temporarily uncomfortable. But this feeling soon passed. The talk turned to lighter subjects, and eventually we parted.

CHAPTER XX

Farewell, Chungking!

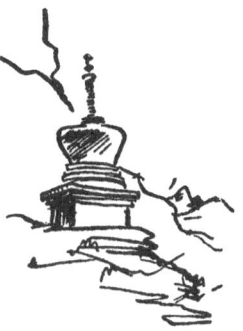

Tibet has always possessed a mysterious attraction for Westerners, and living in Chungking, which in location is almost next door to Lhassa, was a tantalizing experience. It was just as difficult for a Szechuen resident to cross the Sino-Tibetan border as for an inhabitant of Africa or South America to do so.

Occasionally someone from the Tibetan neighborhood would appear in our port, and we would ply him with questions until his mind was squeezed as dry as any sponge. One afternoon a tall, gaunt American clothed in cheap Chinese-styled garments came into my office, and after a brief introduction, asked me to describe the symptoms of diphtheria.

When I had done so, he said, "Yes, that must have been what she had."

Immediately interested, I inquired where this case had been, for Szechuen was not in the usual latitude for diphtheria epidemics.

"At our home near the Tibetan border. My daughter developed a bad sore throat and died. I thought it was probably that disease."

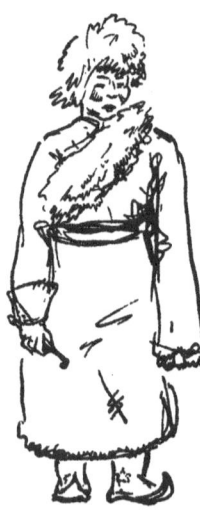

"Wasn't there any medical advice available?"

"None nearer than Chengtu—a three-weeks' journey from us."

"Tell me something about that country," I urged.

He began in a desultory way, but gradually, as the narrative continued, his eyes began to light, his speech came faster, and I found myself listening avidly. His work was among the aboriginal tribes where Szechuen borders on Tibet. Usually he came into contact with the Tibetans only when he made a trip to Ta Chien Lu, the nearest town, and, incidentally, the last outpost between the two countries. Like frontier communities the world over, it had a large floating population composed chiefly of merchants engaged in bartering the products of their respective countries—in this case, China and Tibet. The Chinese name for the town was a key to its activities, for *Ta Chien Lu* meant literally "Big Money Street."

My visitor preferred to talk about the tribespeople; in his opinion they were infinitely superior to the Tibetans and to the Chinese also, though in lesser degree. They seemed to have a good many homely virtues: one of these, honesty, offered a striking contrast to Tibetan thievishness. The Chinese have a saying: "A Tibetan steals until he's forty; after that he turns the prayer wheel."

The aborigines were evidently simple people with very little learning, and, I judged, a most primitive culture. This was why the Chinese had always *chin-kan* (looked lightly on) the tribes and treated them with little consideration. "But they are good and loyal," he defended, "and worth any sacrifice, even my child."

"Your child?" I asked puzzled.

"My wife and I were scheduled to make a trip through the district when our daughter became ill. We went, leaving *Amah* (woman servant) to nurse her, for I had faith to believe that the Lord would take care of the child, and He did."

"I thought you said she died."

"She did."

At the moment there seemed to be no bridge of understanding on which we might meet. It is not my purpose here or ever to criticize harshly anyone's sincere religious belief; also, the unswerving devotion to duty that this man had is a force to move mountains and put most of us to shame. As a doctor, however, all I could see in my mind's eye was the picture of a little girl left with an ignorant native nurse in that lonely mountain district to fight the strangling terrors of diphtheria. Inability to comprehend this "Abraham-and-Isaac" type of parenthood must have flickered in my eyes, for our conversation soon died a natural death. Shortly afterwards my visitor faded from the Chung-king scene, but my brief contact with him made me more determined than ever to see his section of the country.

The opportunity came when I was closing up my work at the hospital preparatory to leaving. A Trade Commission group from the coast arrived at this time in Chungking, with the planned destination of Ta Chien Lu. I packed hastily, chose Lao-mi as personal servant, together with a number of dependable chair-coolies, and joined the party. We had been told that the trip would require thirty to forty days of travel, depending on the stages made. When Ta Chien Lu was finally reached, if any trouble arose, we would have to look out for ourselves, for no government protection could be counted upon.

For days on end we traveled through country much like that of the Yangtze Gorges. While the snowy ranges were to be seen in the distance, a good part of our way lay through foothills and fertile valleys. Later, when the climbing became steeper, we exchanged our sedans for small donkeys. The scenery did not impress me so much as that of the Southwest, but the people were interesting, indeed. These were of three types, Chinese, Aborigines, and Tibetans. The tribes-people were shorter in stature than the Szechuenese; their noses had higher bridges; their hair was long, inclined to wave, and was very oily. We were told that they never bathed in water, using only oil on their bodies, and this none too often, I assumed. They had luxuriant beards, and as these grew, the adornment was rolled up under the chin. In hair and beards, some of the tribesmen had a strong resemblance to the Hindus, but in physique they seemed much closer to Mongols.

Their robes, extending from neck to ankle, seemed to be made chiefly from a sort of hopsacking. Most of them looked as if they had purchased large burlap bags and cut places in these for head and limbs to emerge before wearing them. They wrapped their feet, which seemed very large in comparison with those of the Chinese, in the same sort of sacking and let their attire go at that.

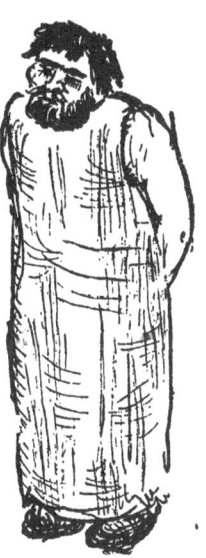

The Trade Commission group halted several days away from Ta Chien Lu, but having come that far, I wanted to complete the journey, and went on alone save for my attendants. The town was much as I had been led to expect, though there seemed to be more antagonism in the air than anyone had mentioned. Chinese, tribespeople, and Tibetans were all out to get the best of one another. No one of these classes had any liking for the two remaining ones. The Chinese looked down scornfully on both; in return tribespeople and Tibetans cordially hated the Chinese. Whatever emotional fervor was left over they used up in hating each other.

Lao-mi and I camped in a filthy little inn, and there one of the coolies brought me a patient. I had to make a chest examination; how this was to be done was a problem. The sacking garment seemed to have no openings, so I took my scalpel and began to cut a slit in the front of the outside garment. Beneath this were others; eventually I counted fourteen in all, though the time was early summer and the weather mild. My patient's body was a rich chestnut in color, but I discovered, with a degree of fascination, that this was not his skin. Inquisitively I began to scrape. The layers of filth and oil came off like softened paint, and when the skin was finally reached, I found it a bilious olive shade, probably due to its never having been exposed to light, or for that matter, to very much air. Remembering that I had thought Chungking filthy, I smiled; in comparison with these people the Chungkingese were immaculate. The Tibetans seemed no cleaner, though they wore robes that were more like garments than these bags.

Since I had to rejoin the Trade group at a certain time, my stay in Ta Chien Lu was limited to three days. I went from one end of the place to the other, and while the sight of a foreigner attracted plenty of attention, no difficulties arose then or on the return journey, which was as uneventful as the preceding one.

Back in Chungking, I finished settling my affairs and boarded a steamer for down river, headed for the Rockefeller Hospital in Peiping and later for similar institutions in Shanghai. After this I was ready to start for home.

Two years or so earlier in Chungking, I had received an invitation one day to the Japanese Consul's residence. At the appointed hour an official chair called for me, and I rode over in state. My host met me in a reception hall and for a minute or two—his English was excellent—we exchanged compliments about the scenery in America and Japan. Almost at once it was suggested that we go in to tea, and there I found members of his family and a number of guests seated on the floor around a low table. All were garbed in kimonos, and without shoes. The Consul was in full-dress uniform but when he sat down, he, too, removed his shoes. I was unpleasantly conscious of my own feet, so I tucked them out of sight beneath me.

Meanwhile, I tried to puzzle out the reason for this invitation. No one seemed to be sick, and when the affair ended I decided that it was nothing more or less than a social gesture.

Two or three weeks later, the real explanation emerged when I was asked to call professionally on the Consul's wife, who was pregnant and in bad condition. The results of the examination put me in a quandary. I considered the treatment she had been receiving all wrong, but anything I did to change it would be experimental. Experience had taught me to move carefully in such matters, so after deliberation, I told the husband what I wanted to do if I took the case, and the risk it entailed. He gave me full permission to go ahead. Luckily everything turned out all right; the wife was delivered of a fine boy, and the proud father was most appreciative of my part in the matter.

When word reached him that I was leaving Chungking, he asked my route to America. I mentioned the hope of going via Siberia, and at once he told me that all arrangements would be made by him between Shanghai and the Russian border. At the time of the offer, I was only too glad to accept this favor; later it proved to have some disadvantages.

The directions were to go straight to the Japanese Consulate-General in Shanghai. There the Japanese entertained me, took care of my luggage through customs, presented me with gifts, and put me on a coastal steamer bound north on the Yellow Sea for Dairen. A terrific storm blew up that night, and rather than spend the night in the stuffy cabin, I borrowed oilskins from the crew and spent a thrilling night on deck, with my chair lashed to a stanchion to keep me from going overboard. The weather had calmed down by the time Dairen was reached. Several Japanese came out in a small boat, escorted me ashore, and after I was settled in a hotel, they suggested that I let them entertain me at a night club. This solicitude was becoming a bit overwhelming, and preferring to spend this evening on my own, I asked to be excused. In the hotel I ran into a British business man I had known in

Chungking; together we set out to see the town. It was, frankly, as tough a community as I have ever visited.

The next day, my Japanese sponsors saw me on the "Chinese Eastern" train which was bound for Berlin, and everything went along smoothly until we reached Manchouli. There we went through the usual procedure of customs and passport examinations, and after an hour's delay boarded our next train. It was summer and everyone was hot, tired, and uncomfortable. When, after advancing for about five hundred yards, the train stopped abruptly and inspectors came through again, exasperated murmurs rose from the various compartments.

Certain that all my affairs were in perfect order, when the officers reached me, I gave them my passport willingly enough. To my amazement, they seemed disturbed, and instead of returning it to me, walked out. Almost at once they reappeared and told me I'd have to get off the train. I protested, insisting on a reason. The one I received was intriguing and, I must say, flattering. It was to the effect that a Russian official had recently been refused admission to the United States because of some passport irregularities, and, in retaliation, they could not extend courtesies to me. After a time I was informed that there was an alternative which would permit me to continue to Europe. It was simply to pay a fine of $56.56, though for what I never discovered.

21

Managing to conceal my feelings, I saw them depart with my good money, and sank back in the seat with only unpleasant thoughts for company. The next moment, the inspectors returned and presented me with a paper to sign. This was a promise that I would spend five dollars gold every day I was in Russia. While I was hopelessly arguing this, for there was not one thing I could do about it except get off the train and perhaps be jailed, one of the officers went through my bags. In the end they walked off with the signed paper and every stitch of clothing I owned, save what I was wearing. They assured me that the clothes would be returned to me when I reached the Polish border. In my mind I kissed them good-by, for I never expected to see them again.

Our route now followed a northwesterly direction, and the temperature changed accordingly. By the time we reached Omsk, the linen suit which I had been wearing at Manchouli was far too thin to keep me warm. In the small basin in the compartment I washed underwear, socks, and shirt nightly. Never having worn rough-dried shirts before, my attire gave even me food for thought, but I was willing to sacrifice neatness for cleanliness.

At Omsk I forgot these minor troubles, for an attractive young woman boarded the train and entered my compartment. When she showed me a ticket to one of the berths, I said, "There must be some mistake—I've been in this section straight through."

"No," she said wearily, knowing her Russia better than I did, "there's been no mistake, but it is possible I can be placed with a woman somewhere, and another man can come in here."

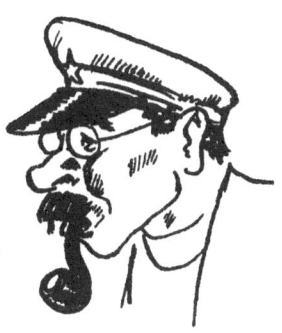

She rang for the porter, and a lengthy discussion in Russian followed. "He says all the women's berths are arranged for and that I must stay in here or get off at the next stop," she told me.

"That's all right. He didn't say anything about the men's berths being filled. I'll get out and leave this for you."

Another argument ensued, and at the close, my new companion gave me a startled look. "He says you are not to leave this compartment—the officials want you to stay right where you are."

Well, I thought to myself, never let it be said that I forced a lady off a train, but right here is where I stop washing my clothes at night, I can see in advance. In a short time we had settled down to make the best of what was assuredly one of the most unconventional of situations.

She turned out to be the daughter of a Russian father and an English mother. Her father, under some political shadow, was working in the salt mines, and she was going to Moscow on business. When we got to know each other better, she confessed her desire to get out of the country but admitted there was not much hope of obtaining permission to do so.

The girl seemed to have very little money. Since I had to spend my five dollars a day on the train and there was almost nothing palatable to be bought in the diner each meal except a fruit compote, I insisted on paying for her portions as well as mine. Warned in advance about food on these trains, I had brought along a small alcohol stove, some ham, eggs, coffee, and several bottles of soft drinks. Why the inspectors did not relieve me of these, I do not know. The water on the train turned out to be so bad that I never even attempted to make coffee, and the soft drinks were rationed carefully to last throughout the trip.

At each stop we got off to stretch our legs. Now that we were in Siberia, the weather was wintry, and my thin suit no protection at all. My companion had a steamer rug and insisted that I use it. Any fashion artist would have found me interesting, I feel sure, as I strode up and down the railroad platforms garbed in a white linen suit and a blanket.

Each of these towns seemed a duplicate of the others just passed. Buildings were all frame, most of them in need of paint, and on each platform were crates of American farm equipment, unused and rusting. The churches in most places were storehouses for grain.

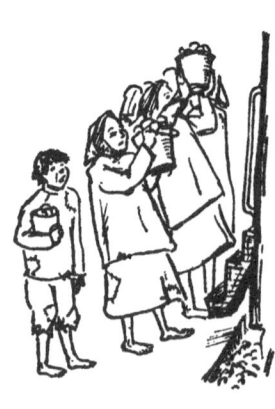

Children, the saddest-looking specimens I had ever seen, huddled in curious groups about the trains, but not once did I see one of them smile or indulge in play.

Crossing the Ural Mountains into Russia proper, I found the land greener and activity greater. Moscow, though, proved to be a disappointment. It was like a great overgrown country town in a dilapidated condition. When I stepped down from the train with my luggage, the porter seized my arm and demanded fifteen dollars gold for his services from Manchouli. Since he had done nothing, this seemed the last straw, but for once the police came to the rescue. A soldier now stepped forward, declared prior rights on my body, and leaving the porter very much disgruntled, led me to the customs.

On the train I had engaged in several conversations with a Middle-European who warned me that for a foreigner in Moscow silence was the only policy to pursue. "Take my advice," he told me, "and do absolutely no talking. It is so easy to say the wrong thing in this country."

Except to answer the customs people in monosyllables, I followed his advice. When they permitted me to take my practically empty bag and proceed, my friend the soldier stepped off with me. People were pausing before a group of pictures on the station wall, portraits of Lenin, Stalin, and others. The soldier now spoke to me in Russian, asking me whose photographs these were. Since I could not understand his language, I did not have to simulate stupidity. He followed this up with English, German, then French, fields in which I was more familiar, but I continued to look blank.

His last remark almost made me give myself away. In exasperation, he shouted in English, "What the —— can you say besides yes and no?" I just walked on, and he followed.

Reaching the post office, I started to enter, but my guard tapped me on the shoulder and gave the signal to move on. Evidently I was too dangerous a character to be permitted in public buildings. At some of the shop windows I was permitted to look in; at others, I was hurried away. This surveillance was becoming much too monotonous. I began circling the telegraph poles along our way, and, to my inward delight, he did the same thing twice.

By that time the fellow had become aware of my effort to make him seem silly, and this venture into the amusing came to an abrupt end. Poking a gun under my shoulder, he told me in Russian to walk the straight and narrow path, or else. At least that was what his tone and the gun implied, and I obeyed. In time I got on the train for Berlin, and at the Polish border we stopped again for examination. Here my bodyguard left me, and to my complete surprise I was given my confiscated wardrobe—but at a price. The Russians had assessed it as excess baggage, and the charge was more than the price of my ticket all the way from Dairen to Berlin. At the moment the things seemed hardly worth the money. Having been handled several times by the Russians and later by the Poles, everything was soiled and mussed.

After Russia, Warsaw seemed a splendid metropolis, and I had only pleasant experiences in Berlin, Paris, and London, observing hospital methods in those cities. When finally I sailed for America, it was with one idea of vengeance—to "smack down" the first Russian I could find in New York. Unfortunately, Russians seemed scarce the few hours I was there, and even if I had met one, I suppose the old influences of law and order would have made me act conventionally.

Later, when I repeated this experience to another traveler, he laughed. "Your being an American citizen was only a flimsy excuse, I imagine. The whole trouble probably started with your Japanese backing. The Russians have made it almost impossible for Japanese to travel on those Trans-Siberian trains, and they have a way of getting all necessary information about tourists before Manchouli is reached. Anyone with Japanese connections such as yours was bound to become a suspect in their eyes."

In those last four hours of my homeward journey from New York to Maryland, I found myself remembering afresh that earlier train ride when I had picked up the pamphlet, and all that had resulted from finding that printed page. Smiling to myself, I recalled the days of preparation, together with my first ardor and determination to scrape scales from the Chinese dragon of traditional medicine. Well, I had worked hard and had created, I believed, some degree of interest in Public Health work throughout the city.

In comparison, however, my influence on Chungking seemed as nothing with that the city had worked on me. I had journeyed a long, long way in thinking since that first disappointed day of arrival. Ugliness, filth, torrid climate—none of these seemed any longer to matter greatly, when I remembered the days and nights in those ancient and mysterious streets. My life had been enriched by strange friendships and by intimate glimpses into the heart of another race. No matter where the path of life should lead me in the future, I should always be aware of Chungking in the background, reminding me that men, regardless of color, creed, or nation, continued much the same as they had been throughout all the long centuries of her history. When everything else was forgotten, when my memories of Chungking's sights and sounds had faded under the pressure of the years, this thought, I realized, would remain with me for all time as a key to the stores of human understanding.